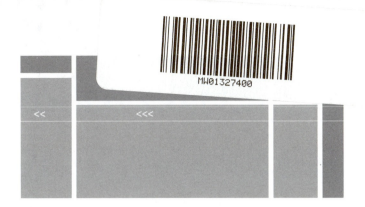

Finding Your Way

A SPIRITUAL GPS FOR CAREGIVERS

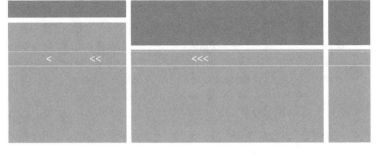

Finding Your Way

A SPIRITUAL GPS FOR CAREGIVERS

SANDY LOVERN

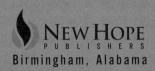

Birmingham, Alabama

New Hope® Publishers
P. O. Box 12065
Birmingham, AL 35202-2065
www.newhopepublishers.com
New Hope Publishers is a division of WMU®.

© 2010 by Sandy Lovern
All rights reserved. First printing 2010.
Printed in the United States of America.
No part of this publication may be reproduced, stored in a retrieval system, or transmitted in any form or by any means—electronic, mechanical, photocopying, recording, or otherwise—without the prior written permission of the publisher.

Library of Congress Cataloging-in-Publication Data
Lovern, Sandy, 1952-
  Finding your way : a spiritual GPS for caregivers / Sandy Lovern.
    p. cm.
  Includes bibliographical references and index.
  ISBN 978-1-59669-246-6 (sc : alk. paper) 1. Caregivers--Religious life. 2. Caring--Religious aspects--Christianity. I. Title.
  BV4910.9.L68 2010
  248.8'8--dc22
                                         2010019391

All Scripture quotations, unless otherwise indicated, are taken from The Holy Bible, King James Version.

Scripture quotations marked (NASB) are taken from the New American Standard Bible®, Copyright © 1960, 1962, 1963, 1968, 1971, 1972, 1973, 1975, 1977, 1995 by The Lockman Foundation. Used by permission.

ISBN-10: 1-59669-246-4
ISBN-13: 978-1-59669-246-6

N094141• 1010 • 3M1

With love

to

My Lord, who took me on a journey
through the darkness and
gave me a burning bush to light my path.
May He be glorified in these words;
Ralph, who was my cup of water in times of
drought;
Jeff, whose unwavering faith in me
beckoned me to the finish line;
Trisha, whose presence centered me
when I strayed off the path;
And to my new extended family,
Chris, the voice of reason for the one I treasure;
Christina, a beacon in the night for the one I love;
and
Alexandra Grace, the hope of a new generation.

Contents

Introduction — 9

Chapter 1: Telltale Signs of the Inevitable:
Tangible Evidence, Surreal Denial — 12

Chapter 2: How Do You Alphabetically File Someone's Life?:
Putting Their Lives in Order — 19

Chapter 3: The Dreaded Phone Call:
You Knew It Was Coming — 26

Chapter 4: The Enormity of the Situation Overwhelms You:
Help! My Loved One Has Fallen and I Can't Get Up — 35

Chapter 5: You Are Not Alone:
This Club Sandwich Has Turned into a Turkey Meltdown — 42

Chapter 6: And Mama Makes Three:
Taking Them into the Fold — 48

Chapter 7: Just a Hint, But a Whole Lot of Hope:
They Don't Know You Anymore — 54

Chapter 8: There Is a Time When You Can't Go Home Anymore:
Time to Lock Up the Old Homestead — 58

Chapter 9: Antiseptic Anxiety:
Hospitals Have Become Home and Doctors—Dragons — 63

Chapter 10: Unraveling Relationships—Learn How to Braid!:
Your Family Is Feeling the Effects — 69

Chapter 11: Looking in a Mirror Darkly:
Where Are All Those Wild Emotions Coming From? — 75

Chapter 12: Pampers to Depends:
Florence Nightingale You're Not — 82

Chapter 13: Delight Their Eyes, Feed Their Souls:
Bringing Home to Them, Wherever They Are 88

Chapter 14: It's Not 30 Minutes—It's 30 Years!:
Visiting Is Taking Its Emotional Toll 96

Chapter 15: Changing of the Guard—You're the Captain Now:
Keeping Family Traditions Now Rests in Your Hands 102

Chapter 16: They Need New Shoes:
Finances Are Stretched, Bank Accounts Diminished 107

Chapter 17: Bacon and Biscuits Beckon You Home:
Sometimes Memories Are All You Have; They're Enough 113

Chapter 18: Where's the Instruction Manual? :
Decisions—You Are Holding Someone's Life in Your Hands 118

Chapter 19: Superhero, Take Off Your Cape—Put On Your Garment of Praise:
Juggling Two Households? You Need Another Hand 124

Chapter 20: They've Changed, But So Have You!:
Did You Ever Think You Had It in Yourself? 130

Chapter 21: It's Time to Take Them for a Walk:
The Signs Are All There—Don't Miss Your Opportunities 134

Chapter 22: Reaffirm, Reassure, and Release:
It's Now or Never 139

Chapter 23: Your Mortality Immersed in a Baptism of Fire:
They're Gone and You Are No One's Child 143

Chapter 24: Two Dimensions, Two Journeys, One Destination:
You Miss Their Essence 149

Additional Scriptures to Give You Direction and Clarity on Your Journey 156
Resources for Caregivers 166
Journal Notes 170

Acknowledgments

Thank you to everyone who contributed to *Finding Your Way: A Spiritual GPS for Caregivers*. The exposure of your raw emotions, ups and downs and victories, will be instrumental in bringing others hope and encouragement, in order to set them free.

To all of the elderly who brought so much wisdom to this work, may your voices be heard loud and clear. To the caregivers, who opened their hearts and honestly expressed their feelings, may your words bring comfort to those who are troubled and heavy-laden.

And for those who have spoken anonymously, thank you for voicing your darkest fears and brightest memories.

I would like to express my sincere gratefulness to New Hope Publishers, who believed in my message and, through print, gave birth to it. Their publishing ministry is instrumental in carrying forth messages from the hearts of God's people, and they are truly the watch guards of His truth.

Then the glory of the God of Israel went up from the cherub on which it had been, to the threshold of the temple. And He called to the man clothed in linen at whose loins was the writing case.
—Ezekiel 9:3 (NASB)

Introduction

<<< >>>

While experiencing the challenges of life as a caregiver to several elderly loved ones, I earnestly sought *wisdom* to address the emotional and spiritual turmoil that altered the course of my family's lives.

Life had taken a turn we never anticipated, and put us on a difficult road we never planned to navigate. For me (I thrive on organization) this threw life into a tailspin. The weight of new expectations that I did not know how to live up to meant putting life on hold. *My* needs took a backseat to others', and I lacked the necessary directions to find the way beyond the enormity of that change.

I desperately searched for something I could latch onto that would make everything all right. My quest took me through massive journals of cold clinical summaries that tell caregivers what to expect medically regarding their loved ones, yet leave the soul and spirit hungry for words of comfort and inspiration. I surfed the Web for a magical formula to turn my chaotic journey into one of sublime peace. I needed to see others' testimonies: personal stories of grace, and vital information from those who had traversed the maze before me and made it through, victorious.

Determined to get into the *minds* of others' loved ones—those who dwell in assisted-living and nursing home environments—I counseled with persons involved in their care. *Somewhere*, I knew there also had to be a place where caregivers could share their mental, emotional, and spiritual anguish as well as guilt. And I found that caregivers' insights provided one key: *care-receivers, our loved ones*, often give us the OK to find a way of peace, if we will pursue that avenue.

Throughout these pages, you will meet a care-receiver—*Mama*—though, in many cases, that name easily translates to *grandpa, father, brother, uncle, husband, grandma, wife, sister, aunt*, and so on. *Mama* is our loved one who engages our memories and emotions, and depicts a person of love, substance, and security in any language, from any neighborhood.

Though not everyone has had a loving parent and pleasant childhood, in light of the best today and future you can have, *Finding Your Way* gives direction to allow you to get around what you wish might have been to what you hope will be.

I pray this *Spiritual GPS for Caregivers* ministers to many of you who are searching for some kind of "godly positioning system" as you go on your way. The life road we travel tears millions of us apart; it's often clouded with emotions and no sign of a bright tomorrow, ridden with hazards and roadblocks, no good change in sight, and no turning back. So the chapters stand alone, to allow you to find what intersects best with where you are on each leg of your journey.

As you read *Mama's* thoughts, I hope you will discover that "her" thoughts may be surprisingly different from your own—and that you will try to leave some of the feelings of guilt and anxiety behind. I believe that the Scripture verses in each chapter—*God's* thoughts—empower you to think past the clouds, obstacles, and hazards as you forge ahead. My prayer is that *Mama* brings you reassurance, relief, a smile, and encouragement along your way. That you find peaceful, golden moments to carry you through your journey. May the Lord—as with everything we encounter in life—show you the peace and answers that you seek. *Godspeed as you find your way!*

Sandy

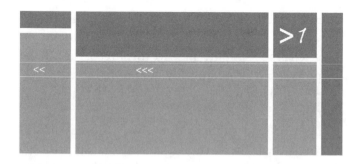

Telltale Signs of the Inevitable

Tangible Evidence, Surreal Denial

And the L*ord* *God formed man of the dust of the ground, and breathed into his nostrils the breath of life; and man became a living soul.*
—Genesis 2:7

EVERY VISIT TO MAMA'S DISPLAYS MORE SIGNS OF trouble, but you try to ignore them. You know what I'm talking about. A strange odor permeates the house and the old piano, adorned with 30 years of pictures, is gray with dust. The bedrooms emit the sour smell of sheets in need of a good washing, and, everywhere you look, there are mounds of newspapers, old magazines, TV guides, and cutout coupons.

What concerns you is the huge stack of bills spilling out of Mama's shoebox onto the kitchen counter. As you rifle through the pile, your heart does a little flip-flop. Past due notices and Mama's grocery list are hidden amongst the thick envelopes holding dreams for the elderly. The dreams are bogus contests offering million-dollar returns to all, if they would "just return the enclosed envelope along with a check." Her checkbook is in the pile, and you glance through it. The once beautiful script that flowed across get-well and thank-you cards is now an arthritic chicken scratch, painstakingly etched across the lines. You realize it might be time for you to take over paying her bills and getting her records in order. That's what scares you, the words *in order*.

In order for what?

You know it's for the time when she will no longer be able to do it herself. The time when you have to make sure her insurance policies are up to date, her will is updated, and her living will is signed. You think maybe tomorrow you will do that, but from the looks of things, you have run out of tomorrows.

The kitchen looks like a discount store warehouse. Mama's once tidy cabinets are rather sticky on the outside and the contents inside are alarming. Boxes of macaroni and cheese housed next to cans of soup, corned beef hash, and tuna fish. Not a vegetable in sight. *Well, Mama always cooks from scratch,* you think, so you peek into the refrigerator. The door discharges a whiff of stale air accompanied by the pungent smell of moldy onions. The vegetable bins are empty, except for rotten carrot tops and dehydrated tomatoes that have been there too long.

Yes, something is going on. Maybe Mama is just not feeling well, having a few bad days. As you tidy up, you notice the garbage can is stuffed with TV dinner trays, paper plates, and candy bar wrappers. The once crisp, hand-embroidered kitchen curtains are yellowed and spattered. The kitchen stove has charred burners, evidence of a fire. That's confirmed as your eyes trail up the wall behind the stove and see a small telltale sign of bubbled backboard and missing wallpaper. *This can be real trouble*, you think, as you envision the house in flames and Mama asleep in her easy chair. Her hearing is not so good these days, and you preaching at her to replace the battery in her hearing aid has gone unheeded.

You stop for a second and remember when Mama's hearing was so sharp. Nobody could ever sneak out the door. No matter where she was in the house, she'd hear that tiny wheeze of the wooden floorboard as you crept down the hallway, or the ping on the screen door that sounded an alarm to her as you pulled it closed.

The drawers and cabinets have roach droppings in them and the salt has hardened in its shaker. Mama loves coffee, yet the cans lay unopened next to the old can opener and a jar of instant coffee sits next to the sugar bowl. *Her arthritis must really be bothering her.* She used to be so fastidious when it came to her kitchen. Every spoon, knife, and fork used to shine in the silverware holder as they lay nestled in a gaily-papered drawer. The old cast-iron skillet that used to turn out the most perfectly golden fried chicken is being used as a doorstop. Mama's biscuit cutter is rusted from sitting in a puddle of water that has leaked out of the flowerpot on the windowsill. You lovingly pick it up and shake your head because you know there will be no more buttery, flaky biscuits cut from it.

Another sign of trouble is the leaking flowerpot. Mama could baby any withered old plant into newness of life just with her patience and love. So why is what appears to be a fern shedding its brown leaves all over the windowsill? And where's the sweet scent of lavender that was as permanent a fixture as Mama herself?

>>> **All the while, you pick up and rearrange things like they used to be.** As you clear off the kitchen counters, you look out the cobwebbed window and see the overgrown yard. The lawn service had guaranteed they would mow whenever necessary, but apparently your connotation of necessary and theirs is totally different. Papa's blackberries are hidden amidst the wild vines climbing up the old fence posts. You cringe, knowing his precious tools are rusting away in the old shed out back.

Huge packs of toilet paper line the bathroom wall. Cans of room freshener sit on the dirty sink, and Mama's teeth are in an old Mason jar, alongside Papa's toothbrush that she refuses to throw out. It's been years since Papa passed away, and yet his clothes still hang in the musty closet. His glasses lay on the sideboard in the kitchen as if he were going to walk through the door any second, sit down, and read the daily paper. Denture cream oozes out of the tube on the counter—*which cannot possibly be sanitary*—and there is a pile of dirty clothes on the floor.

The blaring television is on the shopping channel, and you figure it's never changed since Mama doesn't know how to use the channel changer. The new broom you purchased for her on your last trip is outside the door, still in its plastic wrapper, just like all the gadgets everyone has given her throughout the years. The gifts are all stacked in their original boxes in the back closet.

Your 15-minute drop-by to see how Mama is doing needs to turn into a full-fledged spring cleaning, and it isn't even spring! You can't possibly get started cleaning up the *mess*. You've got a report due at work and *still have to run* by and pay Mama's delinquent phone bill, which is what brought you here in the first place.

Does any of this strike a nerve in you? Helplessness overwhelms you, along with guilt, because you are going to have to leave Mama alone in this mess. You've got time to run out and get her some fried chicken and a new pile of those gossip magazines she loves, and then you have to get back to work.

Maybe she isn't as alone as you think. Papa's presence throughout the house seems to be enough for her. She refuses to leave the old homestead, claiming all her memories are here. Maybe it's because she is afraid, scared that if she leaves, she may not remember anymore. She can navigate the familiar hallways blindfolded, and that security would be gone. Pictures of people she loves smiling out at her would be relegated to cardboard boxes and sealed up, like her life, visited only on birthdays and holidays.

You're caught between two worlds, and so is Mama. You're afraid of what is to come, and she's afraid of losing what's past. Mama is the last person on earth who would want you to worry or feel overwhelmed. She always said she never wanted to be a burden to her kids, but how can you just walk away?

Well, here's some good news. Until you have no choice, and as long as Mama is still able to get around, place your trust in the same place Mama does, in the page-worn Bible that sits alongside her easy chair. She places her life in the hands of the One who knows her every need, far better than you do. Over the course of your own life, wasn't she the one who always directed you to the Lord when you needed strength, peace, or wisdom?

>>> **The guilt that's trying to hitch a ride home with you must be told to take a hike.** *There is no condemnation for those who love the Lord, so seek peace of mind from the Word.* Respect the decisions Mama has made, and believe the Lord for the rest. He will let you know when the time is right, when Mama has gotten too tired to do for herself. But just because Mama isn't baking biscuits anymore, does not mean she is ready to turn off the oven. Give her some time. Let her know you are there for her and keep stocking up those cabinets with tuna fish. *It's so much healthier than hash!*

<<< **Crossroads** >>>

Can you recall a moment when you knew your life, or the life of a loved one, had significantly changed and there would be no going back?

Care Recipient's Response
I woke up one day and couldn't walk, swallow, or use my hands. I was terrified and thought of ways to die. I thought I should have died, rather than be humiliated, but then I remembered my grandchild.

<<<   >>>

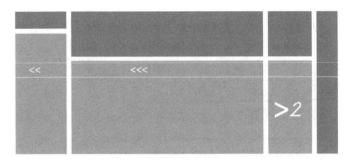

How Do You Alphabetically File Someone's Life?

Putting Their Lives in Order

And also the burnt offerings were in abundance, with the fat of the peace offerings, and the drink offerings for every burnt offering. So the service of the house of the Lord was set in order.
—2 Chronicles 29:35

You've gotten another phone call from the yardman saying he hasn't been paid, and Mama forgot to send a birthday card to your child. *Mama never forgets.* She used to be able to name off every grandchild's date of birth, the year they started school, and every aunt and uncle's phone number. Your to-do list has gotten longer. How in the world can you take on one more project? Right now, your own household demands all of your time. Is there ever going to be a time when you can do all of the things you want to do for yourself?

It seems like your wants are sitting in the bleachers, in time-out, while the other players in life are scoring touchdowns. Then you remember all the times in the past when Mama was there for you, and she needs you now. When you were hospitalized, she was the one who came in and took care of the kids. She forced you to put off cleaning the garage so the two of you could have a quiet ladies' day out. Mama always seemed to call when you needed to have that little extra spiritual push.

Now she needs you, but don't expect her to come right out and ask for help. You can suggest to her that it might be easier if you go ahead and handle her bills while you are also doing yours. Tell her that knowing she is taken care of will set your mind at ease.

Mama has not lost her ability recently to do the things she used to, and she is probably fully aware of her diminished capacity. She's been aware of it for the last 15 to 20 years. Every day that she woke up with a new ache or pain, each time she looked into the mirror and wondered where the beautiful young girl went, reminded her of passing time.

You know what it's like to grow old. You don't need a commercial on television to tell you that aspirin will relieve those aches and pains you have. Every time you bend over to pick up a wayward sneaker, you realize you can't always do what you used to do. This is no surprise to Mama. She has seen these days coming for many years now and is as afraid and irritated with change as you are. By approaching her with the attitude that paying the bills is a project you would like to do for her, she can keep her dignity and some independence.

You've had, or at least thought of having, a conversation with her neighbors, asking them to alert you if there is any sign of trouble; you've talked to the bank to advise them of Mama's condition–now don't you think it's about time you talk directly to her? Make a date to come over for a mealtime get-together. Let her know your concerns. Assure her you are there to help her continue her lifestyle, but there are decisions only she can make, and you need to know what those decisions are.

>>> **Find out where she keeps her important papers and go through them with her.** Yes, those covert documents called *wills* and *living wills*. They're the most needed documents, yet unheeded. They point to a destination all will go. You need to find out what Mama really wants. Her answers may surprise you. Does she want to be on life support, go into assisted-living quarters and when, or make any changes to her will? These are important questions no one likes to ask or hear answered.

You don't want a summons to the hospital one night to find Mama has taken a turn for the worse and the doctors are looking expectantly at you to make split-second, life-defining decisions. It is difficult because you may not have made the transition yet, from being cared for by Mama to being the one who now cares for her. It's a rocky road, and that is why you must have a lot of humor in your life. Yes, it's OK to find humor in the situation. Believe me, Mama wants you to be happy. You're still her child, and like any mother, she wants to see you flourishing in life, not weighed down with responsibilities. She may even have been in the same situation with her own mother or father, but you will never know until you talk.

Communication brings a breath of peace and clarity. You cannot change the final destination of her life, but you can change the circumstances of how she is going to get there. The Bible is where you will get strength and power to do whatever it is you need to do to help. Knowing you have done the best you can for Mama provides you with tools to battle guilt and fear. Prayer can take you to a place of tranquility and resignation. Once you recognize the Lord is in control, all you have to do is be willing to carry out His desire for Mama's life.

You might have the luxury of siblings who will be there to help you, and you might not. Either way, if *you* are there, then you are the one who is going to need to help by doing whatever it takes to make Mama comfortable, and encourage her through this next passage of life. Your whole world is turning upside down, but so is hers. She is aware that things are changing, and will probably have to change a whole lot more before it's all said and done, but that doesn't mean she will be very happy about it.

Mama likes to lull her days away with memories of what used to be because it is safe for her. You are still making memories for your own family, so you feel pulled in two directions. You might be amazed at some of the feelings surfacing in yourself. Before this whole process is over, you're going to find inside yourself that which you never knew was there. Some of what you discover may amaze you, and some may make you feel ashamed. You will find you have great strengths and dark thoughts. It's OK. That is what life is all about—experiencing ranges of emotions, living in those moments, reflecting in them, and coming out on the other side—changed.

Back to business. Organize those important papers, get them signed, witnessed, and put into a safe place. Make sure Mama is aware these are *her* decisions, and promise you'll abide by them. This will give her a feeling of trust, knowing that what she asked you to do you will, in fact, do! When those moments come, and they will, that you have to make decisions, she is depending on you to fulfill her desires, not yours. She must be able to trust you. If Mama says she doesn't want to be on life support, then you must honor her decision. Even though everything inside of you refuses to let her go because you are not ready, this is not your decision to make. This is a decision that's already been made, and your job is to put her wishes into motion.

It is very difficult to follow through sometimes because Mama might not know all the variables you do, but when the final decision must be made, it needs to be hers. You might want to hold on to the last bit of hope, not knowing that Mama has prayed for the Lord to take her home. You might want to believe that any second her condition is going to change, while at the same time Mama is looking toward heaven to release her from her situation.

>>> **What if Mama refuses to allow anyone to help her?** She guards her private papers like a hawk and tries to fool you into thinking everything is OK. Any attempts to help are warded off by disapproving looks and raised eyebrows.

Unfortunately, under these circumstances, you cannot do much. Some people just refuse to allow others to help them. Perhaps they have always been self-sufficient and don't know how to accept help, or maybe they are reacting to a notion engrained in them since childhood that their business is private. About the only assistance you can give, is to let them know, if they ever need help, you will be there for them.

But if Mama is willing, while you are helping her get her life in order, have a nice conversation with her, hold her hand, cry a few tears, and try to keep it light and humorous. I know it's a serious topic, but talking in whispers and averting your eyes, only makes it a fearful situation for both of you. Laughter has a way of dispelling fear, and that's what you want for Mama. So get the necessary things done, file them away, and then spend time reminiscing. Life is still very, very good!

<<< **Crossroads** >>>

How did you feel about someone taking over parts of your life such as paying your bills and selling your home, your car, and other items of independence?

Care Recipients' Responses

It didn't bother me. I knew I needed the help.

>

They were just things, so they were not important to me. I didn't want to go back home after my illness, because my husband was gone and it had now become just a place to live. I wanted to be in a place where people could help me.

>

Everything was OK, since they were just items, but when my car was sold, I felt like someone had died. I loved that car.

>

It was just something that needed to be done, there really were no more choices.

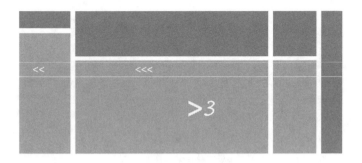

The Dreaded Phone Call

You Knew It Was Coming

And David said to Solomon his son, "Be strong and of good courage, and do it: fear not, nor be dismayed: for the LORD God, even my God, will be with thee; he will not fail thee, nor forsake thee, until thou hast finished all the work for the service of the house of the LORD."
—1 Chronicles 28:20

THE PHONE RINGS AND YOU FREEZE. HAVE YOU noticed that every time a call comes in these days you subconsciously hold your breath? That internal clock is ticking in your mind, and you know logically that time is winding down for your loved one. In fact, it really is only a matter of time. What do you fear when you hear your phone?

You fear the inevitable. It's like a giant looming cloud in your life that you know is one day going to open up and rain all over you. You can't run and you can't hide. Have courage, the Lord is well able to prepare and carry you through this. When the call does come, you are going to find yourself needing to be in constant communication with Him. He will bring clarity where there is confusion, peace when everything seems upside down, and direction when you feel totally lost.

After you receive that call and hang up the phone, a thousand questions fill your mind and fear grips your heart. You wonder how you are going to handle this new situation that has demanded preeminence in your life. Appointments need to be canceled, trips diverted, finances rerouted, and dreams set aside. Immediately, you muster up your strength to act like David, facing your Goliath. You tell yourself you can handle this, it will only require a little rearranging of your life.

Most people are doers. As long as they can be doing something, they feel they are going forward, and that's a good thing. But sometimes busyness is used as a means to push back or ignore our emotions. Only you can judge your actions. If you find yourself mixing up a batch of brownies at midnight while at the same time rewinding the tape of your Spanish lesson, then you might discover that you are trying to use work as a diversionary tactic to avoid what is really bothering you.

God is a God of order. If you aren't sensing peace inside, now would be a great time to ditch the brownies and replace the Spanish with some good old prayer. Having a conversation with the Lord, and asking Him to bring order to life brings peace. Holding onto His hand reminds us He is in control of our situation.

Over the next few days, weeks, or years of Mama's life, you are going to get very familiar with some extremely powerful feelings that have the ability to strengthen or destroy you. Armed with the Word of God, knowing how to pray, and wait on His answers, equips you for the battle ahead. Whatever your present knowledge of the Bible, dig in and find out the promises He has for you and your loved one. Simply talk to your heavenly Father who is always ready to listen.

The direction of your life may have shifted, but it is only for a while—a season. You can look at this time as an opportunity to rise to the occasion, or you can look at it as a burden. Now is the time to stop and make some conscious decisions of how you want to approach your new life. You can't ignore the situation or control it, so what do you do?

You can accept the new call placed on your life! Make a commitment to the Lord, your loved one, and yourself, that you are going to do whatever it takes to finish this race. Step out in faith with no road map, no guarantees and no provisions, and believe He will provide a cloud by day and a fire by night to lead you just like He did the Israelites, when they were wondering in the desert.

How's Mama handling all of this?

>>> **She's reeling with a thousand emotions herself.** Her entire world is changing, and she knows that her race will be different than yours. Hopefully, she's already set her eyes toward an eternal home, while you see visions of graduations, children's birthday parties, and grandchildren yet to come. You are both looking forward, but with different endings to your

journeys. Your job is to mesh those two journeys, and grab all the memories, smiles, and hugs you can along the way.

You will get past doctors' difficult diagnoses, depressing nursing home faces, and the worrisome days by making the most of the time you have together. Humor helps so much, though it may seem out of place. Mama wants to see you smiling, and if that's what makes you both feel better, then try to keep smiling.

What if Mama is too demanding? There might be instances when Mama can, and will, abuse the situation. She will have you hopping around like a bullfrog after a dragonfly. There are limits to everything. You also have a family, job, and your life. How do you tell her no and not become immersed in guilt? Know yourself and your motives; works do not measure love. If you have Mama's best interest at heart, then you know your motives are pure. How you find balance will depend on your circumstances.

Mama does understand the difficult position you are in, and there are decisions she also needs to make. You did not create this situation, and you can't change it. You will need to find a solution that will work for the both of you. Mama may want you at her bedside every night at nine o'clock to brush her hair, but you also have bills to pay, maybe kids that need help with homework, and a husband or a wife, who needs attention, as do you. It is all about compromise and what you can live with.

Your emotions are going to try to run your life, so constantly turning to God's Word helps set them straight. Your soul will run you ragged with these emotions, and the only way to control your soul is to submit your spirit to God. Communicate with the Lord. Get alone with God through quietness and meditation, and let Him sift through all the emotions. Although Mama's voice can get very loud in your head and heart, sense His voice and Word dominating the situation.

Mama was always there for you. Your mind will pull you back to a childhood school recital and flood you with joy as you remember Mama clapping. You see that smiling face as you planned your wedding and hear the voice that gave you strength as you complained about the baby keeping you and your mate up all night. So what do you do?

>>> **You make Mama's life as comfortable as it can possibly be.** Surround her with items she loves, spend uplifting time with her, and then focus on your family and needs. You cannot live Mama's life for her, nor can you make it better in her own mind. Let's face it, the elderly can sometimes behave like irrational spoiled children. They've lived a long life, possibly a difficult one, and may feel they've earned the right to some of their bad behavior. If you have an 80-year-old who wants watermelon, but the doctor says he or she can't have it, are you going to deny it to him or her? Weigh everything and then sometimes let the heart override man's wisdom.

If watermelon goes against medical recommendations, then you have choices to make. I can almost guarantee, either way you decide, guilt will be there to greet you. The key is to make choices that leave no regrets. If you decide to only see Mama three days a week instead of seven, can you live with that? Don't let your decisions be made from a guilt perspective, because Mama will sense that in you. She doesn't want to be a burden to you. Don't devalue her existence by visiting her just because it seems like the right thing to do. When you do visit Mama, make those visits count.

Create a scrapbook you can both look over, or read together from books by favorite authors. If there's a wheelchair, move around inside the residence or venture outside. Feel the sunshine together and listen for the birds. Make the world bigger than the building's walls where she lives. It doesn't have to be a big deal; simply make your visit more than going and clucking over her situation and staring at the television with her.

Plan something enjoyable. If you make the times you share memorable, then it gives Mama something to anticipate. More is not always better and it does not make you a more dutiful child. Sometimes your loved one wants to look at you. Seeing your bright smile and laughing eyes reassures them that when they are gone, you are going to be all right.

If you begin to feel deep resentment, it is time to pull back and reassess what you are doing. It is natural to feel some irritation; your ordered life has become quite chaotic. But if that irritation resides long enough, it will develop into resentment and bitterness. At that point, you will be unable to help your loved one. Bitterness will spoil every area of your life. Do what you can for your loved one and then rest in that. If he or she isn't handling the situation very well, or if they are demanding more than you can give, that may be something they are going to have to work out for themselves.

>>> **Communication is vital for a healthy relationship.** Don't be afraid to ask Mama to tell you how she is feeling. Encourage her to tell you the things that are bothering her. It may be something as simple as she doesn't like the way the nurses brush her hair, or she might not like the way they talk to her. There are a lot of little things you can do to dispel her anxiety. There will also be some issues you can't fix. Nothing is better than talking to one another and sharing your feelings.

Mama has known you your whole life. Do you think she has forgotten how much you hate hospitals or doctors? She knows you are a very reclusive person who loves your alone time. She understands how important your children's school affairs are to you, and she realizes her situation has changed, but your life has not. Talk over these issues with her; she is still Mama. Some concerns may surprise you and seem very trivial, but remember, Mama is still a human.

The elderly know they are not as attractive as they once were, but they still want and need to be touched. Their often liver-spotted, gnarly hands want to be held, and their furrowed brows need to be kissed. Old age scares us, and we sometimes think of our loved ones as breakable, porcelain figurines. With those thoughts, we subconsciously put them on a shelf, only to be touched on rare occasions. Touch has healing powers within itself.

Go ahead. Push Mama over in the bed and climb in there with her. *These are the moments to remember.* Infuse her with the heat and warm Spirit of your body. When you have left her for the day, she will still be thinking of you, snuggled up next to her. When

Mama is gone, these are the kind of memories that will sustain you and relieve that old monster called *guilt*.

>>> **So when the phone call comes for you, be ready.** You have been thinking of this call for a long time now and, when it comes, it is almost a relief. What you have been dreading has now occurred, and you find it really isn't as bad as you had anticipated. You've got some immediate changes to make, and the rest will unwind before you. Be reassured you can handle this situation, and when times get so dark, remember it is just life evolving. It happens to everyone and the only thing different in your case, will be how you react to it.

You are not alone in this; others are watching you. Children, no matter what age, do see everything. How you handle yourself will have a big impact on them. You might not see that influence for years to come, but you will eventually. Your commitment to your loved one is called a *long-term investment*. Whatever portion of your life you invest in the care of your loved one, will come back one hundred-fold in your own life.

As your children see the respect and honor you give your loved one, they will in turn give back to you when you grow old. As a parent, you never abdicate the role of teacher. You are tenderly caring for Mama just as she cared for you. You picked up your loving traits from someone. When you were small, Mama was teaching you, and you didn't even know it. Can we smile now? See, the circle of life goes round and round and round.

<<< **Crossroads** >>>

What do you dread the most in the family caregiving process?

Family Caregiver's Response
The daily grind of the care. No matter how hard you work at care giving, the patient continues to slide south. The reality is, there is nothing you can do but work harder every day.

What advice would you give others going through or about to go through the same process?

Family Caregiver's Response
Be strong, as there will be emotional times that you will have to address. You will make it. Just continue to put one foot in front the other. Give the best care that you can, and I promise, there will be no regrets.

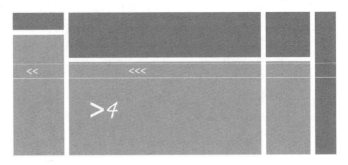

The Enormity of the Situation Overwhelms You

Help! My Loved One Has Fallen and I Can't Get Up

*Then was our mouth filled with laughter, and our tongue with singing: then said they among the heathen, The L*ORD *hath done great things for them.*
—P*SALM* 126:2

THERE COMES A TIME WHEN THOSE YOU LOVE BEGIN to lose their agility and decision-making skills. The situation can sometimes become stifling and overwhelming. It seems no one around can make a decision, and you're bombarded with needs all day long. You find yourself longing for those carefree days when the hardest choice you had to make was what color nail polish to put on or where to go for dinner.

Your mind develops a direction of its own and it always seems to want to lay basking on a hot tropical beach or sit contentedly on a porch listening to the cool rain as it pelts the tin roof overhead. Your thoughts want to be anywhere other than closed up in a hospital room or conscientiously counting out the correct dosage of pills.

Your patience is stretched way beyond its limits, and if one more person asks you to do something, you will pack your bags and leave. *To the ocean—and maybe even an oceanside condo—here I come!* Your family doesn't understand why you always retort so sharply, and your siblings, who have neglected to help in the care of your loved one, have the nerve to tell you to chill out. Ugh!

Does it make you feel any better to know there are thousands of people in your situation? Well there are. And every one of them is thinking the same thing you are...that they should be able to handle this, but they're having a very difficult time doing so. It's that old black cloud called guilt, which by now has learned how to control your thoughts and thereby dictate your actions. The key is for you to get a hold of those thoughts and master them.

How do you do that? You open up your Bible and replace your thoughts with God's thoughts. They have the power to override human wisdom and thrust you into the spiritual world where God lives and moves. Have you asked Him what He has to say about the whole situation? You will be surprised to find He thinks you are doing just fine. He knows your limitations and, let's face it, this is a huge emotional ordeal you are going through, and from the looks of things, it could go on for some time.

Why wouldn't you be upset seeing your loved one's slow demise before your very eyes? This is your mama we are talking about! You remember Mama folding clean dishtowels, and now here she is wearing them as a bib while you spoon-feed her tapioca pudding.

>>> **Give yourself a break and allow yourself to fall apart occasionally.** It is OK to do that. You are experiencing many brand-new emotions, and you need to own them. If you are afraid, call upon the Lord who tells us to fear not, for He is with us always. As you spiral to the depths of that fear, see yourself on the other side, victorious in His power. The worst thing to do is ignore or suppress the emotions you have. That's called *denial,* and it results in you not being present in that moment. If you keep looking back, you will miss the time you have today with your loved one. If you keep looking forward, you're not present today. I'm not saying to stay in those dark places, but you must travel through them to experience the saving power and light of the Lord.

We've been conditioned to turn the table of blame on ourselves. There is always something more we should have or could have done. Why is it blame always has to be placed somewhere? It's not your fault Mama got sick, the dog decided to eat a chicken bone out of the garbage can, or your computer chose today to purge itself. Your family does not miss those home-cooked meals as much as you think. So what if the ceiling fan is whirling spider webs into the air. Realize that you are subconsciously making huge decisions every day. If you have sought the Lord in your daily devotional time, then you must believe you are being led by His voice.

There comes a time to relax and trust, and it is a very difficult thing to do. As Christians, trust is the basis of our relationship with a Savior we can't see, and we sometimes find out we have been fooling ourselves with our professions of faith. Be honest with yourself. If you are one who naturally likes to control, then it will be extremely difficult for you to reach that elusive place called peace. A good starting point is to believe He lives inside of you, so begin by believing in Him.

Put your trust in the choices you are making because if you don't, you will be laden with guilt for years to come, and that is one heavy companion to tote around on your back. If you have to make the decision to put your loved one in a nursing home, or get them assisted living because you need to keep your job, then believe God will handle the rest. Never forget that the loved one you have had the pleasure of spending some beautiful years with really belongs to God. He is still the one responsible for all of our lives. Take off that huge weight you have been carrying and lay it at His feet.

We all tend to have the attitude that if we don't do something, then it won't get done. To a degree that is absolutely true, but it is the extent you carry those thoughts that can, and will, make a difference in you and your loved one's life. Mama wants to see you happy, and she can sense when you are tense and out of sorts. If your family, co-workers, and even animals can sense your energy, don't you think she can? We tend to think our loved ones have lost their ability to feel deep down inside because they are older, or not as alert as they used to be. The young woman who diapered you is still there, she's just the one now wearing the diaper. The football fanatic that used to huddle with you in the yard is still there, he just doesn't recognize his buddy.

So how do you keep your energy sweet?

There is something you can do and it is well worth the effort you put into it. The first thing in the morning, take time to be alone with the Lord. He will give you the faith, direction, comfort, and strength you are going to need to get through just one day. Faith is not like bottled water that can be stored up and poured out when you need it. It is an active force that must be refilled every day. The faith you had yesterday that Mama was going to be OK will not be enough to carry you through today as you look at her inability to get out of bed.

>>> **Avoid the martyr syndrome like the plague.** I'm sure in your life you have seen people whose faces are lined with bitterness and their conversations are laden with long sighs. You can avoid the syndrome by remembering you are the one who has been entrusted by the Lord, to fulfill a promise He made to your loved one, or their partner.

Try looking at your situation in this light. Your loved one might have been married and previously lost their mate. Think about that for a moment. Their mate might have prayed that the one they love would always be taken care of by the Lord. Since they are gone, it is up to someone else to fulfill that promise. You are the eyes, ears, hands, and feet of the Lord. You are the one making their bed, baking up tasty morsels to entice their appetite, and making huge decisions regarding their life. Consider it an honor.

The Lord looked at all of His options and then His eyes fell upon you!

As always, the Lord has a way of turning everything you think you are doing for someone else, into something that is really benefiting you in the long run. You will not see it for years to come, but it's all there. Every time you place a steaming hot cup of tea into your loved one's tired hands, or struggle to pick them up from where they have fallen, you are pouring yourself into their lives.

So when you find yourself flailing on the floor with Mama, or shaking your head over one more thing that has to be done, turn your eyes toward heaven and call for help. He will reach out of the heavens, pluck you up, and give you the supernatural strength you need to become the person of faith He has called you to be.

<<< Crossroads >>>

What did you discover is the most important thing in your relationship with your loved one, and what will you remember the most?

Family Caregiver's Response
In the early stages of her disease, my mom and I would laugh and talk about the past. I knew her mind would fade and that time would never return, so I took advantage of it. When I look at my mom today, she is my hero. As I look into her eyes, I see my mom from the past, the good and fun times we had, not as she is today with the disease. I was lucky God blessed me with such a great mom.

Care Recipient's Response
When I was 25 years old, my stepfather passed away, and on his deathbed he asked me to take care of my mom. I never forgot this. When you are a stepchild, you never appreciate your stepfather until he is gone. When I became a father, only then did I understand. I hope he is proud of me now.

How do you see yourself? Young, in love, a new bride?

Care Recipients' Responses
In my 30s, young at heart, and doing things with my friends.

>

Wrinkled, my skin looks like a prune, and at this age, an old woman.

>

Not 30 and also not an old man.

<<< >>>

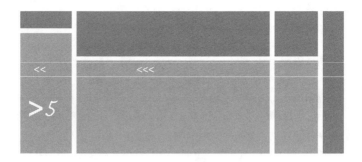

You Are Not Alone

This Club Sandwich Has Turned into a Turkey Meltdown!

My heart panteth, my strength faileth me: as for the light of mine eyes, it also is gone from me.
—PSALM 38:10

THE PRESSURES ON TODAY'S HOUSEHOLDS ARE tremendous, and when you add caring for a loved one on top of them, they can sometimes seem insurmountable. It is a lonely place to be, and one where it appears there is no one to counsel or guide you. Who do you talk to that can give you advice and guidance? I'm talking about someone who can listen with a caring heart, because they have also been there. You don't need any more lists of agencies that provide services, you need someone who will tell you it's not going to be easy, but you are going to get through it.

You'd be surprised to know that there are thousands, just like you; you've just not heard about them. The statistics are alarming. Due to better health care, seniors are living longer. Our elderly population is rapidly growing, and the number of people financially able to take care of them is dwindling. According to the US Census Bureau, there are 35 million people over the age of 65, and that number is expected to double by the year 2030. By 2050, there will be more than 82 million seniors over the age of 65. Seniors over the age of 85 are the fastest growing portion of the US population.

Statistics are boring but they are instrumental in painting a realistic picture of where you are in the whole scope of things. According to the numbers, you are right in the middle of where you are supposed to be. It may not make you feel any better, but it is always good to know you are not alone. Interestingly, we seem to function better in tough situations, knowing we have others stuck in the same hole.

Look around the office where you work, the church you attend, or the grocery store. Talk to people and you will find so many others just like you, caring for their loved ones, unsure of what to do for them, and afraid of losing them.

If you were lucky enough to have been born between 1946 and 1964, then you have earned the title of baby boomer. But this generation has also been honored with another title called the Sandwich Generation. It is an official title *Merriam Webster* added in July 2006. If you have not heard of this title yet, or don't understand the significance of it, the term means those individuals who are wedged between two worlds. They have aging loved ones and are struggling with the predicament of also having a family of their own and possibly dealing with grandchildren, siblings, or friends who are ill.

You also have a special month, called Sandwich Generation Month, which is annually celebrated nationwide in July. The month was designed to bring awareness and education and to also commemorate those who are caring for the elderly. Statistics show that more than 1 out of every 8 people between the ages of 40 to 60 are raising children of their own and taking care of an elderly parent. Those who are caring for an aging parent from a long distance, weighs in at between 7 to 10 million.

National Family Caregivers Month, celebrated in November, is a time to thank, support, and educate the 65 million family caregivers in our country. Research and see if you can find some activities going on in your community where you can connect with others in your situation. A support group of people who understand what you are going through is always helpful. They may relate some of the things they did, to help get them through the caregiving process that you can utilize in your own situation.

You may be so tired you can't even comprehend all of the above figures, but if you can get the gist of what they represent, then you're going to be able to get a handle on the enormity of your situation. The figures will not change your life or bring your life back to what it used to be, but they are your present reality. Knowledge brings understanding, and though it can't answer all of your questions, it does give some substance to your new role.

When you look at the numbers, there really is very little escape from the situation for anyone. If those you know are not right in the middle of what you are, then they've already been there, or it looms large in front of them. This journey has no U-turns or detours. You're on a path and you might as well get the best directions you can, which means information and communication.

All of this will not alleviate your tiredness or your discouragement when you have to deal with your loved one, but know there is an end. This journey you are on is a one-way street and you had better prepare yourself for those bumps in the road.

>>> **One way to prepare is to make sure you take care of yourself.** Get rid of that old thinking that tells you you're being selfish or self-centered. If your motor breaks down, you are not going anywhere, and you sure won't be able to give anyone a ride. Take time for yourself. Get plenty of rest and pamper yourself every once in a while. To continually do a job with no reward only brings discontentment and apathy.

It is OK to take the afternoon off and go see a movie. Splurge on a lavish lunch or dinner and see how quickly it revives you. It brings you back to "center." Taking a moment for yourself gives you time to reflect and evaluate what things are most important to you. And for dessert, have a big helping of the Word. It has sustaining powers within itself and will nourish your depleted soul.

The last thing you want Mama to see is you having a meltdown. So take some time to replenish yourself, and then you will have an abundance to pour into her. You've got to find the little nuggets throughout this journey, and I'm talking gold here, not some fast food you pick up on the journey. Remember that lavish lunch? Check, please!

<<< Crossroads >>>

What advice would you give others going through or about to go through the same process?

Family Caregivers' Responses
I can no longer enjoy rounds of golf with my father, go out for lunches or dinners, or watch football games...all these things are "gone," although my father is still here with me. This is all very difficult to take. Advice: join a support group, and make time to visit your loved one regularly.

>

Make sure their financial affairs are in order and you have a power of attorney. Have a long-term care policy.

>

When you are placed with your back against the wall, you can do some amazing things.

What seems to be the most difficult times for the residents, and is there anything family members can do to make it better?

Professional Caregiver's Response
Holidays. And if you can't be there, send flowers or something special. They share it with the whole building, and it is somewhat of a competition in their little community. They love to show off.

What is the one, single most important thing a family member can do to help themselves and the residents adjust and live with the situation?

Professional Caregiver's Response
Become a part of where they are living. Call them or the facility, email caregivers, and they will read your messages to your loved one.

How well do residents adjust to their new surroundings, and what makes for a good transition?

Professional Caregiver's Response
It fully depends on the family. If they were dysfunctional before, the relationship with their loved one does not change. Happy families that communicate, have very little problems, whereas those whose loved ones used manipulation and moodiness to get what they want will continue that behavior.

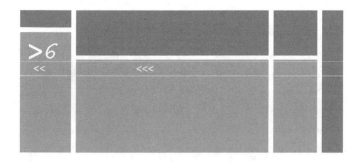

And Mama Makes Three

Taking Them into the Fold

As an eagle stirreth up her nest, fluttereth over her young, spreadeth abroad her wings, taketh them, beareth them on her wings.
—Deuteronomy 32:11

YOU HAVE MADE YOUR DECISION THAT RIGHT NOW the best place for Mama is with you. Well, the situation you see her in has really made the decision for you. It all sounds good as you mentally make the move in your head. Since the kids have gone off to college, there is that spare bedroom; you can move the extra television in and squeeze Mama's easy chair into the living room. Everything appears to be doable physically, but have you considered how the change will affect the dynamics of your life?

Unless you mentally prepare yourself, you might find yourself challenged beyond what you had anticipated. You are not bringing home an adorable puppy, you are bringing another person into the cozy confines of your nest, and it takes a lot of preparation. You can make the adjustment a whole lot easier if you rearrange your thinking, before your rearrange the furniture.

How you do that depends on what type of person you are. Some people are logical thinkers, and some people are creative dreamers. First of all, to make the move a smooth transition, be honest about what kind of person you are, and don't stray from your own reality. If you are a logical person, then you should probably set up some kind of methodical system that works for you. If Mama likes to have her coffee as soon as she wakes up, and your morning routine involves whipping up lunches, feeding the dog, and cleaning the bathroom counters as you brush your teeth, then it might be better to get Mama into a different routine.

If you are a creative person that likes to fly by the seat of your pants and Mama wants to watch *Jeopardy* every day at 6:00 P.M., then you might want to invest in some kind of recording device. In other words, even though Mama is moving in, she is not going to, and should not be allowed to, take over your home. Get rid of the feelings that you are being unkind. You are being realistic. You're already in a new situation, and the least amount of change you can get away with, the better. Muster up some backbone, because you are the one who needs to stay on an even keel. If you start to take on water, the whole ship is going to go down.

There is a way to make the transition good for both of you, but it takes time to find that delicate balance. We can't forget it's also a huge change for Mama. She is moving into an intimidating atmosphere and leaving behind everything familiar and dear to her. It's intimidating because it is the unknown, and she might feel threatened that the little independence she has is being taken away from her.

When someone else enters another person's space, there is always opposition. It is merely the way we are designed, and this does not mean you do not love Mama and want the best for her. You will also feel a little threatened. Your space is being invaded. What you feel is a natural response to the situation. Don't make the mistake of shying away from your own feelings. Make sure everything stays "real." Own up to what you are feeling, and ask the Lord how to temporarily relieve the feelings of frustration you're experiencing.

>>> **There are other members of your household the change is also affecting.** Your husband may be entirely supportive, but his support does not take away the irritation he feels of having to share the love of his life with someone else. Your children now have to tiptoe around and be sensitive to Mama's needs. As long as everyone realizes there are some unwelcome changes happening, then you can discuss and deal with them openly.

Mama does not want to inconvenience anyone, but until some adjustments are made, her moving in will inevitably create some chaos for a while. In the meantime, there are many ways you can make Mama feel welcome. First of all, make sure she has her own space. You can do that by surrounding her with things she loves and assuring her that though things may appear to be a little intimidating, in time they will work themselves out.

You can move the bed to allow for Mama's wheelchair and buy a special pan to poach her eggs in, but what can you do to lift the oppressing air that seems to reside in your home now? Laughter ringing through the house has turned into the clanging of the walker coming down the hall. The ambiance once created by your soft candles and cinnamon scent is negated by the harsh smell of disinfectant and soiled sheets. I'd love to tell you to just rise above it all, but that is not your reality right now. So what can you do?

This is where you will learn the true meaning of empathy. *Merriam Webster's Collegiate Dictionary* (Tenth Edition) says that empathy means "the action of understanding, being aware of, being sensitive to, and vicariously experiencing the feelings, thoughts, and experience of another—of either the past or present—without having the feelings, thoughts, and experience fully communicated in an objectively explicit manner." That's a mouthful, but what do all of these words mean to you?

It's the adage, "walk in another man's shoes." It has to be enough for you to look at Mama's face and see her joy at feeling safe with you. When you see her sitting in a chair, hair brushed and a clean nightgown on, versus the condition you found her in, understand you are making a difference in her life. Most importantly, you are helping her keep her dignity. These thoughts should give you what you need to make a whole lot of allowances, for the things you are missing right now.

In days to come, you will once again have your house all to yourself, and then you will yearn to see Mama contentedly sitting in her easy chair, munching on popcorn with the family. What will carry you through the hard times of missing her will be the satisfaction you have in knowing you did all you could for her. Because you did what was right in the sight of the Lord, you won't have to deal with the guilt so many carry. I didn't say it was easy; I said it was right.

As the Scripture above says, your nest is being ruffled and completely disrupted. You will find yourself fluttering around, carrying a huge amount of responsibility on your shoulders, but you can handle it. You are experiencing what it feels like to spread your protective wings and carry someone who is weaker.

So open your heart, and your front door, to Mama, and make her feel welcome. She is bringing so much more than suitcases into your home; she's bringing a wealth of history and a whole lot of thankfulness!

<<< Crossroads >>>

Do you understand how your children and family feel about you having to move out of your own home? The guilt they are going through and the anguish of wanting to give you the best they can to see you experiencing a good life? Is there anything you'd like to say to reassure them you are, and will be, OK?

Care Recipients' Responses

I'm satisfied. I don't want to live with my children; let them have and live their own lives. My own mother did not take care of things, but I have learned from that and want to make it easier on my children.

>

I'm happy where I am; and I try and let my son know that so he can feel good about the situation.

>

The children should have no guilt; it's just a time in life where there are no choices.

What is the most important thing a family member can do to make the transition pleasant?

Professional Caregiver's Response

Make sure their loved one is part of the decision-making process. Surround them with items from their home. When you go shopping for them to move, take them with you. Ease into the decision by beginning at home with communication about the changes to come.

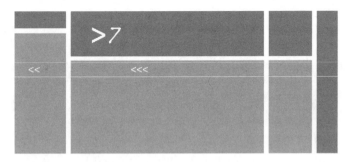

Just a Hint, But a Whole Lot of Hope

They Don't Know You Anymore

And it came to pass, that, when Elisabeth heard the salutation of Mary, the babe leaped in her womb; and Elisabeth was filled with the Holy Ghost
—LUKE 1:41

FOR THOSE WHO ARE DEALING WITH LOVED ONES WHO can no longer recognize them, there is no more sharing of memories, or smiles of acknowledgment when they enter a room. It's as if someone has pulled a shade down, and there is nothing but darkness.

>>> **Your loved one is living in a world you can't enter.** Each time you visit, you feel the small stirring of hope arise in anticipation that maybe today will be the day they remember your name.

It is very difficult to come to terms with your situation when there is very little communication with the one you love. You mull over in your mind the thousands of things you wanted to say when they could have understood them. You wonder if your presence makes any difference at all, and you have a hard time dealing with your emotions that hunger for a familiar touch.

Mama is still there, she has just gone to a place you can't define. Think of it as a woman who is carrying a baby. She has never touched the child, seen its face or heard its cry, yet she is very much connected to the life inside of her. Her baby lives in its own unseen world where it hears, senses, feels, and moves. Just because the baby can't communicate with its mother or those around it does not negate its existence or presence. As the Scripture above states, the baby heard Mary's voice from within the womb, and leaped for joy.

The embryonic sac is paper thin, yet it might as well be a concrete wall. No man enters into its mystical sphere, yet a human being lives and breathes just inches from a human's touch. It's as if two worlds are simultaneously existing side-by-side.

That is where you are with your loved one. They may be physically sound and within your reach, yet you can't unlock their mind or heart. Their condition baffles medical experts, and until someone can find the key to open up their minds, you live in hope. Hope that one day you will see a glimmer of remembrance, a spark of recognition, or a flicker of the person you used to know.

The Bible tells us that we and the Father have become one, but we can't physically see any difference. How many times have you wanted to reach out to touch the face of God, and your hand clutches nothing but the wind. Paul tells us, "I am crucified with Christ: nevertheless I live; yet not I, but Christ liveth in me." He could not see Christ, but he felt His spirit, and that's where you can connect with Mama.

Your journey is a little more difficult than some, because you need to move in a higher state of being. Your reality has already bypassed this worldly realm, and to reach the one you love, you must step out in hope, which is the blueprint of faith. You press on in love and cannot allow yourself to be moved by what you see. Believe that your love has enough power to transcend the walls that encompass your loved one. Trust that your faith has the power to move past Mama's unresponsive flesh, into the very marrow of her bones.

>>> **Let your hope lie in faith that Mama is living in her own world surrounded by your presence, love, and faithfulness.** Besides, we know for the One who can raise the dead and walk on water, Mama's mind presents no obstacles for Him. Believe Him to provide everything your loved one needs, and give Him your faith to work with. Never give up on the miraculous power of God. Every time you visit, go expecting a miracle. You never know when that sparkle of recognition will shine.

can you just walk away from all those years? What's going to happen to the house? How is she going to take this? It's all she has, and this is where all her memories are. How can you do this to her? Do any of these questions sound familiar to you?

There are a lot of things happening at once, and it will take you some time to sort through all of your emotions. The thought that this is absolutely final, probably sends you reeling. Mama will not ever be going back home, and your forward destination is filled with unknowns. Looking back, home represented a safe haven for you, even if you only visited once or twice a year. It was a solid rock that never changed, as boring as you used to think it was. Well, in reality, Mama was the rock. It wasn't the house or the old tire hanging from the oak tree. It was Mama, always ready to give you some advice, encourage you when no one else would, and love you even when you were unlovable. That is essentially what you are turning the key on. Now, Mama is not able to be there 100 percent for you like she used to be.

>>> **You can almost look at it like a rite of passage.** You are truly all grown up. You can't blame your loved ones now for any part of your life because all the decisions are yours. You are totally responsible for everything, including Mama.

Think about how Mama feels. She isn't there to see you turn the key one last time, but the day she was taken from her home, she felt what you are experiencing right now. The difference is, her memories did not flood her tired mind, they trickled in, calming her nervous anxiety.

As you picture Mama racing through the yard to tend to your bee sting, you remember the strength she always possessed. Mama sweetly remembered your vulnerability as you toddled across the floor and your first childhood hurt that she couldn't make go away.

You both experienced powerful emotions as you savored the memories of the old homestead, but there comes a point when you have to face forward. When the future looks dim and uncertain, hope is a tremendous force to draw on. You're hesitant because you don't know what is around the corner and it's so much easier to stand still. You know where you've been, but moving forward brings a whole lot of doubt and fear. The thoughts keep coming. *Why did this have to happen? Mama deserves better than this. If I close my eyes, maybe I won't see Mama's anxious face looking at me for all of the answers.*

For those who may not have had loving parents or an ideal childhood, closing the door of the old homestead may bring a sense of relief. It is another chapter of their life coming to a close, and a long awaited one at that. Some have childhood homes that contain dark closets and suffocating walls. Now is the time to rise above the memories that are holding you back, rejoice that all things pass away, and behold, all things become new.

>>> **You can't change what was, but you can take a deep breath and look toward the heavens for advice on how to handle what is coming.** If you purpose in your heart to do the best you can for your loved one, it will bring you a tremendous amount of healing and wholeness.

You may be turning the key on your old life, and the road ahead may look bleak, but you are going to find some amazing moments along the way. They won't be light-up-the-sky memories, but they will bring you great comfort knowing it was the tiny, sweet moments that made Mama so happy. So, turn the key and toss it.

Lot's wife looked back toward the city, because she was drawn to what used to be and unsure of what was ahead. For her actions, she was turned into a pillar of salt. When you see no road ahead, it's difficult to step out in faith, and even harder to let familiar things go, but faith is what He requires of you. Set your face forward and don't look back. If you will just trust Him, you will discover He has great things in store for you.

<<< Crossroads >>>

For a family member struggling with the inevitability of having to put their loved one in a nursing or assisted living home due to physical limitations, what one thought would you tell them to alleviate their guilt and sorrow?

Care Recipients' Responses

Make peace with yourself. It's for you and your loved one's benefit. Taking care of a loved one at your own home…it doesn't work. Don't blame yourself.

>

Ask God for help. Everything depends on Him, and if He calls me tonight, I'm ready to go home.

>

I've been happy. People need to adjust to where they will be living. If they adjust, they will enjoy life.

<<<   >>>

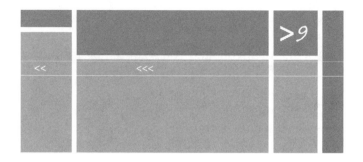

Antiseptic Anxiety

Hospitals Have Become Home and Doctors—Dragons

Multitudes, multitudes in the valley of decision: for the day of the LORD is near in the valley of decision.
—JOEL 3:14

IF YOU ARE NOT THERE YET, A TIME IS COMING WHEN your loved one will probably be hospitalized. There is no way to prepare for this because in the minds of most people, hospitals are very hostile atmospheres.

When those glass doors slide open, you are immediately overwhelmed by an antiseptic odor. And I don't care how great your makeup foundation is, the florescent lights make everyone look sick. Sitting in a waiting room, you are surrounded with people you don't know and not many of them have cheerful expressions on their faces. You are already afraid, so as nurses briskly walk by and doctors authoritatively enter, you resort to an almost childlike behavior.

>>> **You feel like you have little or no control** and are at the mercy of the hospital staff. Since they have more knowledge than you, and you want the best for your loved one, you tend to sheepishly look at them to tell you what to do and when to do it.

There is nothing natural about standing next to Mama's bed and seeing her body fluids flowing out of her and a medicinal cocktail flowing in. There are unnatural sounds echoing down the icy hallways, people moaning, coughing, and calling for help. The hospital chairs are a far cry from your recliner, and the clanging of meal trays is unnerving.

The hospital staff does try to make things as comfortable as possible, but they are there to do a job. They rattle off a list of Mama's medical conditions that you need a medical dictionary to understand as they snap down the bed guardrails and dial up the IV. The doctor briefly stops by and gives you a short, and I mean short, synopsis of how serious Mama's condition is, and then almost taps his feet, as he waits for your response.

You are expected to make medical decisions for your loved one that could determine whether they live or die. Who can do this? Medical technology has come a long way, but the heart of man has not changed. We were never designed to make a lot of the decisions modern technology is forcing on us. Who can decide if a loved one should get a feeding tube or a respirator? Mama told you she didn't want heroic efforts made to save her life, yet the doctor says she needs the feeding tube to get stronger. But if her medical condition does not improve, she will not softly pass away; she will live for years, simply because she now has a feeding tube.

Where is the line between your loved one's wishes, your wishes, and the Lord's? You will need to make some very hard decisions, and without the help of the Lord, you will never be able to make them. He will give you all the wisdom you need when you ask, but you have to be willing to hear His answers. Sometimes we want our loved ones to stay with us forever and don't consider the fact they may have already made some decisions.

I'm sure you've heard that many people die when no one is around. Could it be because they finally feel free enough to leave? I wonder if looking at our sad faces as we surround their bed doesn't create an anxiety in them. They are worried about those they are leaving behind.

So how can you get through the tough times ahead and lessen the anxiety for yourself, and your loved one?

Make absolutely sure your loved one has a living will that explains what procedures they want, and don't want, at the end of their life. This is their job. Your job, is to follow through with their desires. That's the hard part. You want them to stay at all costs, and they want to go. Think about this. They are fully trusting that when the time comes, you will honor their wishes. That does not mean they left the decisions in your hands, it means you are to enact the decisions they have already made. It is not an easy place for anyone to be in, but you can make it through this.

>>> **And there are ways to make your hospital visits easier.** Make friends with the staff who are caring for your loved one. If you have a loving and cheerful attitude, it will make it much easier for the staff, and they will bend over backward to help you. These are the ones you have entrusted your loved one to, so give them praise and support for their skills and the dedication they have for their job. Many in the medical field are Christians, and they face unpleasant situations every day, so be that breath of fresh air for them.

Decorate the hospital room with little items familiar to your loved one. It might be her comforter, a picture, or his Bible. If your loved one is incoherent, don't let that stop you from communicating with him or her. Her spirit or his spirit is very much alive, and humans never relinquish the need to be touched and loved.

Be prepared for the doctor's visit by having pen and paper available so you can write down what is said. Don't be afraid to ask questions, and if you feel the doctor is being too pushy, or not taking the time you need to comprehend the situation, gently explain your feelings. You are the only one who can speak for your loved one, so let your loved one's voice be heard. You don't want to have guilt feelings later with those "you-should-have-asked" thoughts.

You do have certain rights, and so does your loved one, so familiarize yourself with them. Knowledge can bring a sense of peace and control for you. You should know what are the acceptable practices for the situation your loved one is in, and if you feel they are being slighted in anyway, speak up.

With the Internet so available today, it is hard not to begin a medical quest on your own when you hear certain medical terms. That can be a good or bad thing, so let the Lord lead you on this one. Sometimes having too much medical knowledge you don't understand can hurt you. You read about something on the Internet, and suddenly you feel like an expert on it. If you have chosen to be a self-proclaimed medical private investigator, present your questions to the doctor as an inquisitor, not a prosecutor.

Decisions, decisions, so many in the valley of decisions. The next time you visit the hospital, look around and ask the Lord to open your eyes. You carry the Word, a precious commodity inside of you that not everyone has. Ask Him to use you as a vessel of hope to others around you who are faced with similar situations but lack the vital tool of faith. For those like you, who are caught in the valley of decisions, you can be the one who breaches the gap for them between this world and heaven.

Hospitals are tough situations to be in, but if you remember everything is just for a season, then you can muster up faith for one more day. And that is how you will make it through all of this...one day at a time.

<<< Crossroads >>>

What were you feeling when things were discussed such as your living will, what kind of medical treatment you wanted, and where you wanted to live?

Care Recipients' Responses
It didn't bother me. I thought it was a necessary thing.

>

I haven't done it just yet, but my bags are packed to go.

>

I felt very comfortable talking about it.

Were you excited about the changes to come or discouraged?

Care Recipient's Response
I was excited about getting out of the nursing home and going into assisted living quarters. The first night in my new apartment I looked at all of my personal items surrounding me; pictures, my own space, and then I cried. I felt happy and safe. I was glad that I had finally made a decision and was settled.

<<<   >>>

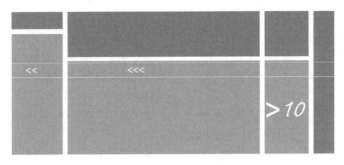

Unraveling Relationships— Learn How to Braid!

Your Family Is Feeling the Effects

And if one prevail against him, two shall withstand him; and a threefold cord is not quickly broken.
—ECCLESIASTES 4:12

ALL OF US HAVE A PLACE WITHIN OURSELVES WE CALL "normal." It's a place that makes us feel all is right with the world even though the toast gets burned, the dog has chewed up another pair of shoes, and the mortgage is behind. With all the mishaps, it is still your life, and one you have control over.

But what happens when the responsibility for someone else's life is suddenly thrust on you?

Before, it was so easy when you could just run by, take Mama out to lunch, and make sure her grass was cut. You know Mama is eating frozen dinners, and you yearn to walk in and smell her beef stew simmering on the stove. You see her feeble hand reach for her coffee cup, and you think if you wish hard enough, you will see it strong again, braiding her grandchildren's hair.

>>> **You will experience a tug-of-war within yourself on this journey you have never sensed before.** As your life begins to unravel you will probably catch yourself constantly reaching back into your memories, trying to recapture what once was, and is no more. It's the "what is no more" that can trip you up. If you don't learn to adapt and accept the new changes in your relationship with your loved one, you could find yourself constantly ensnared by feelings of anger and frustration.

To add more to your already heaping plate of must-dos, there is also the changing relationships in your own personal life. If your husband is dealing with an ailing mother or father, then like it or not, there are feelings that will surface which will surprise you. When your mother-in-law's needs become paramount in your husband's life, and you think you have become a secondary thought, there can be all kinds of mixed signals being sent off. And yes, even in times of sickness, our good and bad emotions will rise to the surface.

Your spouse may be totally supportive of you spending all of your time with Mama, but it does not dispel the feelings he or she has, that he or she is just a tad neglected. There may even be anger, but realize, it is an anger at the situation, not at you or the loved one. As long as we are human, we will have beating hearts that get hurt and very creative thoughts that sometimes lead us into troubled relationships.

We can be very manipulative as humans if we so choose to be, and this is something to guard against.

If your husband is caring for his mother, don't burden him more by trying to get him to choose between you or her. That is a lose-lose situation. You may get him to forgo his nightly visits to his mom, but all you will get is a man consumed with guilt as he sits across from you at the restaurant.

>>> **This journey you are on will require a lot of compromise and a whole lot of "I'll-pay-you-back-later" promises.** There may be wedding anniversaries spent in fast-food restaurants after spending the evening in a hospital, or your cozy pizza and movie nights may be replaced with washing sheets and giving Mama a bath. It is very difficult to watch the man you love bent over with fatigue after hearing another discouraging doctor's report. All you want to do is grab him and run as fast as you can back into the wonderful world you used to have.

You struggle with wanting to make allowances for his mentally shouldering the responsibility of his loved one, but you also want him to understand your feelings. So how does everyone operate who are involved in these new circumstances? Whose emotions should be considered first, and what situation demands priority attention? As strange as it may seem, these questions will come up, even if they only surface in your mind.

When you have a night out planned and your husband feels the need to stop by the hospital or nursing home, how are you going to react?

Right now, your reality could be encapsulated into one huge word, *responsibility*. Ugh, did you feel the heaviness descend upon you as soon as you saw the word? This is just a microscopic view of the pressure you are operating under. It is stifling and will sap every bit of energy you have unless you build yourself up and stand on the promises of the Lord. Make a decision to be one whose demeanor and actions cause your family to rise up and call you blessed, one who merits praise from your spouse and family.

Sometimes, no matter how well you think you are handling things, your family may appear to be unraveling. If you have children at home or in college, the whole family will be rocking when Mama, who used to be a quiet force in their life, now appears to be demanding center stage. Because of diminishing finances, your daughter's dream prom dress has been downsized, and your son's college football tickets are a luxury you can no longer afford. Your well-deserved vacation has been put on hold, and your husband's golf membership is threatened.

Besides financial worries, there is the time element that can't be ignored. Your evenings are relegated to seeing that Mama's needs are met, and, as your laundry mounts up, your patience diminishes. You have to constantly make choices, and no matter how efficiently you organize your time, someone or something is going to get neglected. For those who were once the center of your universe, there is going to be some hurt feelings. In all this confusion, you are going to have to soothe a lot of ruffled feathers, while still plumping Mama's pillows.

You may be asking yourself if you are up to the challenge. Be reassured that if you are the one called upon to juggle the lives of others, then the Lord has equipped you with all you need to do the job. You just have to find that fine balance to your life.

It's there, and you will find it as long as you are not expecting your perfect life to flow as it once did. For a time, you are going to experience some rough waters as you navigate through this emotional and physical process.

>>> **When the stress threatens to overtake you, call upon the One who calmed the waters.** His voice still has the power to make the seas subside and the winds cease. So, close your eyes, take a deep breath and count to three. Remember, a three-fold cord is not easily broken, and if He is entwined in your life, you can stand against whatever comes into your life and be victorious. So, batten down the hatches against the winds of life, and hold on...His help in on the way.

<<< Crossroads >>>

Do you have any advice for others going through the same situation?

Family Caregivers' Responses

This situation puts a severe strain on families. This has not been easy. Once my mom has passed, I have a lot of making up to do. My goal is to take care of the special one in my world the rest of her life. She never asked to put herself ahead of my mom, and I thank her for this. We have both put our lives on hold, and I know God will bless us for this.

>

I'm sure the patient's attitude plays a big part. If they are just miserable, is there really anything a family member can do, or is it all up to the patient and their decision to either accept the change or not?

Professional Caregiver's Response
No! Family members cannot do anything at all to change their loved one's attitudes. Some people are miserable and nothing will ever make them happy. They have to adjust and enter into the place, wherever they live, and accept it as their reality.

Is there anything a family member can do to change the resident's perception?

Professional Caregivers' Responses
Communication is vital. Immediately, get rid of nursing home perceptions. Don't force your loved one into something just to alleviate your guilt. Think of it like leaving a child in kindergarten their first day. You want to protect them, but ultimately it is something they have to do on their own. They will be OK, so you just need to walk away.

The type of person they were at 30 is the same type and attitude they will have when they are 85. They don't change. They are adults that have lived a full life already, you have not. They are stronger then you think. Be realistic, what are your options? Wean yourself from them. Adjust and go on with your own life. You have just changed your loved one's place of living and made their life better. They are now safe, clean, and healthier.

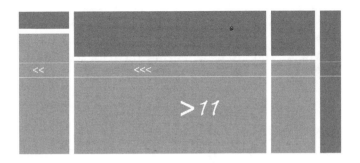

Looking in a Mirror Darkly

Where Are All Those Wild Emotions Coming From?

For now we see through a glass, darkly; but then face to face: now I know in part; but then shall I know even as also I am known.
—1 Corinthians 13:12

Through this whole process of caring for Mama you are going to experience emotions that one moment reduce you to tears, and the next, bring you great joy. All of your own methods of managing your household were thrown out the window the day Mama went for a midnight stroll through the neighborhood in her nightie. And your weekly planner is no longer an agenda, it's a reminder of what was once your way of maintaining some form of normalcy in your life.

Is it any wonder your emotions are erratic? And no, you are probably not going through menopause or a midlife crisis. Besides, being low on estrogen or testosterone isn't the villain that is dredging up those astonishing feelings that keep surfacing out of nowhere. You are experiencing the dark feelings no one wants to talk about and absolutely no one will own up to. I'm sure you have confronted a few of those ugly thoughts and wondered where the pit was they arose from. You didn't believe you could have some of the thoughts that whiz through your mind. I say whiz because they are so out of the realm that we normally think in that no one wants to spend any time entertaining them.

Here are a few examples of thoughts that may have surfaced, and the list could go on and on:

> I can't do this anymore. Mama is going to have to go into a nursing home because I can't stand anymore oozing sores, dirty diapers, dribbling during feeding time, or the constant smell of sickness.
> I love her, but sometimes I wish God would take her. It would be better for both of us.
> Why can't she at least try to help herself? Doesn't she see I am exhausted?
> I don't want to waste another day of my own life, playing nurse.
> I just want my life back to normal.
> I want my spouse and children back. I don't want to keep juggling all of these lives.

It seems so bad when the thoughts are actually verbalized, doesn't it? Would it surprise you to know that many others have these same feelings? You are not alone, nor are you a terrible person. You're tired, discouraged, and fearful. You're caught up in something you never wanted or planned for.

When these emotions arise, we tend to feel ashamed of ourselves and a little fearful that we could even contemplate such thoughts. The soul is so deep, and it is not until times of stress or fear that the hidden heart of a man is revealed. Don't misunderstand the message here. The thoughts do not reflect how you truly feel; it is the mind's defensive way of flight from a situation.

Think of the enormity of what you are facing. It is natural to want an escape from the decision-making process and the inevitable passing away of someone you dearly love. But unless you have the anointing of Elijah, you will not be praying down rain or telling dry bones to rise up. You can see Mama through this if you have some tools or resources to work with. You will not come out on the other side unscathed, but with your battle scars, comes an amazing breadth of grace and wisdom, along with the ability to look back and say, "I did it!"

>>> **Arm yourself with the Word of God, and wage war over the battlefield of your mind.** When each thought comes, catch it and replace it with the promises of God. This may sound trivial, but it is an extremely difficult thing to do. If you don't think it is hard to do, just try to clear your racing mind right now for 60 seconds. It requires the same discipline as maintaining an exercise program, and we all know how challenging that is to do.

If you can gain victory over your thoughts, it will make you victorious in all areas of your life. Replacing your thoughts with the Word of God establishes Jesus and His Word as Lord of your life, not just Savior. Let Him help you control your thoughts, and then you will have control over how you are going to react to situations.

Research the Scriptures and find the ones that speak to your heart. Find a few that you truly believe in, and when challenges come your way, pull them out of the repository of your heart. They will become your sword in the spirit.

Once you have your Scriptures, it's time to get a bigger vision than Mama lying in a hospital bed. By a vision, I mean a small goal you can work toward and attain. For some, the goal may be seeing Mama sitting up, comfortably watching television. For others, it may be getting Mama involved in creating a new life for herself by encouraging her to join some craft classes, or meet new friends at the nursing home. It all depends on your loved one's physical and emotional abilities.

Lessen the stress and expectations you have for yourself by starting with small attainable goals, like seeing Mama covered with her favorite blanket, bathed, powdered, and watching television. You may not be able to do a lot of things to make Mama's life any different, but you can do this! If you'll release your unattainable expectations and congratulate yourself on simply making Mama comfortable, then you can rest, knowing you have done your best for her.

When thoughts begin to bombard you, condemning you for all of the things you haven't done for Mama, remember to mentally reach for your Scriptures and wage war over your mind. Blame is very prevalent in people who are caring for loved ones, and if you let it, it will steal every small victory you achieve. In your mind, there is always something more you could do and even more you didn't do. Somewhere you have to draw a line and rest. You can literally drive yourself mad and overwork yourself so much, that you become useless to everyone around you. If you set some inner guidelines within yourself, they allow you space to breathe and peace for your mind.

When those dark thoughts come creeping in, don't take them personally. Yes, I said personally. In other words, think rationally. Check yourself and your motives. You know that if there was any way in the world you could change the situation, you would. That being the case, your motivation is good, not driven with evil intent. Don't get caught in the quagmire of thinking that deep down inside you are really a bad person. Reject those thoughts!

>>> **Laughter is a great way to battle those dark thoughts.** When those foul emotions bubble up, laugh them away. If you harbor the thoughts, they will negate all of the love and hard work you have invested in your loved one. Sinister thoughts that are not immediately dealt with, will turn your labor of love into a struggle to validate your love.

You may be thinking, *Well, that is easier said than done*, or *You have no idea what I am faced with*. OK, you just did it again. You took the thoughts and dwelled on them. Right now, laugh out loud. Sitting in the midst of all your problems, laugh. And if you can find absolutely nothing to laugh about, laugh just because you can. Savor the life coursing through your veins, the strength to go on one more day, and the hope of better days to come.

>>> **Humor is important.** Yes, it is a serious situation you are in, but walking around with a long face and your eyebrows raised in frustration is not going to change anything. You can expend energy on finding something more to worry about, or you can use that same energy on trying to find something humorous in your recent experiences with your loved one.

Think back to when you tried to prop Mama up in the shower and you both got soaked, or when you had to capture your loved one as they paraded down the corridor in their diapers. Find the humor in the changed relationship you both have. If you don't, they will immediately sense it and acquire feelings of guilt themselves. They will begin to feel they are a burden, have robbed you of your life, or have lost their usefulness.

Laughter has a way of diffusing a situation and bringing light where there is darkness. The Bible speaks of laughter as medicine, and this is one dosage you don't have to check with the doctor about. Arm yourself with the Word, get a vision of what you can truly do for your loved one, and then pour out a spoonful of laughter. Just as in childbirth, the Lord has a miraculous way of taking painful experiences and transforming them, by using memories that were created throughout the experience. When it's all said and done, you're not going to remember the medical dilemmas, you are going to remember your loved one's look of thankfulness, and hopefully there will be a little laughter too.

<<< Crossroads >>>

What brings you the most joy from the caring process?

Family Caregiver's Response
I get satisfaction from spending time with him just walking and talking with him. I feel very content after visiting him when just before his bedtime I am able to attend to his bedtime duties; changing him into his PJs, bringing him a nighttime snack/treat, tucking him under the sheets, and turning on his music for him to fall asleep with. When I leave him to go home, I feel a certain amount of sadness, but at the same time, I feel joyful because I was able to make him feel more comfortable.

If you could have done anything different, what would it have been?

Family Caregivers' Responses
As I went along this journey, it took time to learn about the disease. I wish I had had this knowledge up front.

>

I have no guilt about something that I feel should have been done any differently.

>

I would have taken my mom to see the doctor myself when she wasn't feeling good a year ago instead of relying on her to handle it.

Professional Caregiver's Response
Don't wait. Make decisions while loved ones can participate in the process. Do it while it is a choice and they have the ability to make that choice versus a have-to.

<<<   >>>

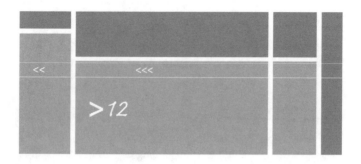

Pampers to Depends

Florence Nightingale You're Not

Naked, and ye clothed me: I was sick, and ye visited me: I was in prison, and ye came unto me.
—Matthew 25:36

JUST WHEN YOU THOUGHT YOUR GOLDEN DAYS WERE within reach, you find you are clipping coupons for adult diapers. Your world has been turned upside down, and you find you are not dealing with it very well. Along with the physical challenges you are faced with, you also have to deal with some pretty murky emotions. You have always been a caring, compassionate person, yet when you are faced with a full diaper or a drooling face, you feel anger and resentment rise up.

Quit beating yourself over the head, and calm down. Overnight you have not lost your salvation or turned into an ogre. Say hello to life, and embrace all of the emotions the Lord has given you. You could not feel such anger at the condition of your loved one, if you did not have such love. You wouldn't cry for their lack of dignity, if they didn't stand so tall in your heart. There is no devil ruling and reigning in your heart, exposing the real person you never knew was there. You are just dealing with life, and that includes the whole expanse of what you are made of.

No one wants to see the woman who threw a wedding together in three weeks reduced to one who is unable to organize her bills. This is the same woman who modestly covered her knees and refused to wear a pair of pants, and now she is naked and trembling in the shower, exposed before you. You hate that it has come to this, and you are trying to find a way of escape. Mama needs you right now, and you must find that mysterious place inside of yourself that you never knew existed. It is a place that empowers you to do what you have to do, whatever that is. You won't know for months or years to come, where you ever got the strength to do what needed to be done. But there will be a day when you will look back and be amazed at yourself. At that time, you will understand that only the Lord could have given you the strength you needed, and then, you will be in awe of who He is.

In the meantime, how are you going to get through all of this?

Understand that the feelings you are experiencing have nothing to do with how much you love your Mama. You remember everything she did for you, and you would move heaven and earth for her. It's just hard to change those urine-soaked sheets one more time. You cannot escape the fact that you are human. Certain things aren't pretty, no matter how you disguise them. It is a special breed of people who nurse and tend to the elderly. We can't all be painters, writers, bankers, or farmers. God has instilled in each and every one of us special gifts, and when we have to move outside those boundaries, we feel uncomfortable.

Here's an example. You may be an expert at math, so you have no problem taking on Mama's bills and insurance forms. Those are your skills, and you are good at them. You don't do well with changing diapers, but your sister the nurse doesn't miss a beat when it comes to diapering Mama. You cannot measure your love for Mama by what you can or cannot do for her. Your love was formed through the daily relationship you had with her over the years. You can't equate spoon-feeding her with her feeding you as a baby. It makes logical sense to correlate the two, but in reality, they are totally different. This is Mama, your stronghold, the one you run to with problems, the one who has always been there for you. You don't quite know how to be there for her yet, but you will.

What if you are caring for someone who never gave you much love or support? How do you deal with those wild emotions that make you want to walk away, and leave them to their own demise? You know, those dark thoughts of *You made your bed, now lie in it*. Remember who you are and the spirit that now lives inside of you. When Christ came into your life, He made His home in your heart. The reason you can rise above the past is because when you were born again, old things past away and all things became new to you. If feelings of anger still linger, let Him bring restoration to you.

Caring for the unlovable or ungrateful is very difficult, and will require you to dig deeper inside of yourself than you may have ever done. Your final objective is to leave behind a legacy of a life lived through the power of Jesus Christ. Remember that others are watching you. Your children, friends, and family are observing how you handle what seems like an unpleasant and impossible situation.

>>> **Instead of trying to convince yourself everything is OK, deal with where you are.** This is your reality, so try to find a way to make some kind of sense of why this is all happening to you. Throw out your preconceived ideas of what you should be feeling, and open yourself up to let God show you what He expects from you. It is very important how you handle this area because it will color everything you do. You want your memories of Mama to be sweet ones, not ones darkened by stained diapers and sorrowful eyes staring at you.

You may be embarrassed about the thoughts you are having, and afraid to tell anyone your true feelings. It can become so unpleasant at times, you may want to load up your car and drive to destinations unknown. You'd like to leave all of the decision-making, problems, and drudgeries behind, in hopes that when you return, life will be back to normal. Like a bad dream, maybe when you come home, Mama will be humming in the kitchen and making her mouthwatering biscuits.

How do you deal with something you don't even want to face?

You deal with it through the counsel of the Lord. He knows every hair on your head, and only He knows how to make it all right for you. Ask Him how to turn the task ahead of you into something that will honor you, Mama, and most of all, Him. If you never moved as a servant of the Lord before, you are about to become a hand servant of His. You're going to be the enactor or fulfiller of all the promises He made to your loved one. If you can grab a hold of this mindset, you will find you can do unbelievable things in His name. You'll be empowered from on high with a strength that would make Samson envious, and you will have an endurance that will remind everyone of the little engine who kept sputtering, "I think I can, I think I can...I *know* I can."

<<< Crossroads >>>

What do you dread most about the caring process?

Family Caregivers' Responses

When we have to change my father as one would change a child, it is a very humbling and sad situation.

>

That Mom expects one of us to be there every night, even though there are health-care workers to help her get dressed. It makes for a long day, and she doesn't even care.

What brings you the most joy about the caring process?

Family Caregivers' Responses

Knowing that my mom is at home rather than a nursing home.

>

On occasion, after tucking him in bed, I say good-night and he will look up at me with a somewhat childish stare and tell me thank you. I am not sure he really knows what he means when he says that, or perhaps he really understands the situation and is truly grateful.

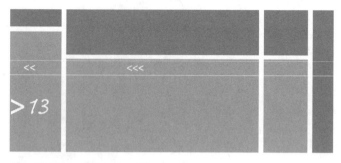

Delight Their Eyes, Feed Their Souls

Bringing Home to Them, Wherever They Are

In the multitude of my thoughts within me thy comforts delight my soul.
—Psalm 94:19

I'M SURE YOU'VE HEARD THE SAYING, "HOME IS WHERE the heart is." That is so true. If you've ever sold a home or gone back to visit the house you grew up in, you realize it isn't home to you anymore. You may have nostalgic feelings of playing under the old oak tree in the front yard, but as you look around, you no longer have that comforting feeling. You know your Mama is not in the kitchen making meat loaf, dad is not tooling around in the shed, and your family dog is not sitting at the door waiting to greet you.

Your presence and the things you surround yourself with are what make a home. Take a second and look around the room you are in. What do you see? Maybe you are sitting in your comfortable chair reading this book with your favorite afghan draped over your knees, Grandpa's heirloom clock is loudly ticking, or you might see pictures of your loved ones and the smell of coffee reminds you it's home.

It's not the place so much as the objects you love to see, touch, hear, and smell. You can help your loved one by surrounding them with items that stir their soul. They might not be able to remember who you are, or even to respond, but their soul is very much alive. Look around Mama's house and see what she has placed next to her bed, atop her dresser, or next to the chair where she watches television. These are the items you should pack up and bring with her. Change is unsettling for any of us, but it is especially difficult for the elderly and those who are ill. They don't have the ability to change gears as fast as you do, but given time, they can change.

>>> **The idea of surrounding Mama with her treasured items is really just good-old common sense.** When mom is not around, babies do better if you swaddle them in something that carries her scent. Puppies thrive when you put an old piece of your clothing in with them while you are away. Why? Because scent comforts us and makes us feel safe. Have you ever been stopped in your tracks because a smell caught you and lured you back to a memory you hadn't had for years? Scent is a powerful tool you can use to bring your loved ones emotional comfort, wherever they are.

Search for items you know Mama has worn continually or placed around herself. It may be an old bathrobe, a ragged nightdress, or an old patchwork quilt, but whatever it is, don't negate its importance. Your initial thought might be to go out and get Mama all new items in hopes it will bring her joy. Your intentions are good, but they are not what Mama needs right now. You've seen babies who hold on to security blankets and the reason is, they love the touch and smell of them. I'm sure you have a favorite pair of old jeans or sweatpants you wouldn't part with. It's the same theory. Mama wants to touch what's home to her. Let her keep that wrinkled old nightgown. If it looks too bad, get her a new robe, but don't make the mistake of replacing things that are dear to her.

>>> **Surround her with pictures of her loved ones, decorate the walls with drawings from her grandchildren, and stimulate her with news of the family.** Unfortunately, as we go about our daily lives, we tend to forget our loved ones are still living theirs also, they just may not be as full as ours. Even though they are enclosed within four walls, they still want and need to be informed of the outside world they exist in. Read the newspaper to them, even though it might seem like they can't hear or understand a word you are saying. Try writing a journal together. It not only puts order and some structure to your visits, but it gives your loved one something to look forward to.

There are so many things you can do to make your loved one feel valuable and a part of your life, while at the same time wrapping their own world around them through their senses. Be creative!

What if you are not a creative person and that old logical mind keeps marching back to the basic needs?

Here are a few ideas you can use. Some of them may have to be modified to fit where Mama is living.

Decorate with plants. Just having something green and alive in a room brings life and energy into it. A fish tank is a great idea because it brings movement, color, and sound into the stillness of life. A bird is low maintenance, and it can become a great source of companionship when people are not around. If your loved one is able, it's a good idea to give them something they can take care of. This gives them a reason to get up every morning, and also provides them with a sense of purpose. We all love to know someone needs us, and a pet might fulfill that need.

If your Mama was an avid crossword puzzle worker, get some crossword puzzle books, enlarge them so they are easier to read, and do them with her. This will stimulate her mind and also provide an avenue of conversation. As much as we hate to admit it, those visits with our loved ones can sometimes be very stilted and boring. What do you do for that long hour? If you take the time to make some plans, then you will find yourself looking forward to your visits.

To overcome the antiseptic odor of hospitals, bring sweet scents into the room. Fill small sachet packets with Mama's favorite fragrances and put them under her pillow. Spray her nightgowns with perfume so when she lays her head down at night, she can smell something familiar. Remember, Mama is still a woman. She loves to feel feminine and probably needs it more now than ever before in the disinfectant world she is living in.

Another great idea is to take a large picture frame and get pictures of your loved one that cover the expanse of their life. Make a collage of the pictures and hang it on the wall. It's a wonderful way to honor your loved one and the life they have lived. Pictures also are an interesting way for the staff to become familiar with them. Snapshots bring a humanization to the patient-hospital staff relationship.

After you have surrounded Mama with things she loves, the rest is up to her. You can create the ambiance, but only Mama can make the decision that it's enough for her. She also needs to make some adjustments because you do still have your own life to live.

A long time ago, your loved ones made their own decisions that are directly affecting their lives today. They may have chosen to live and die in the town they were born in, and you have now moved hundreds of miles away. Though you have pleaded with Mama to move closer to you, she has refused. You can't feel guilty about not spending enough time with her. If she lived with you, or 20 minutes away, you know you would be seeing a lot more of her. Let that guilt go.

Think about your loved one's life. Think about where they live, the family, and friends they have surrounded themselves with. All of these things were of their own choice, not yours. Everyone is entitled to a life of their own design. You have also orchestrated a life by choosing where you want to live and the people you want to surround yourself with. As harsh as it may sound, it is not up to you to change everything you've created, in order to take care of your loved one. What you can do, because you love Mama, is make her life the best it can be, taking into consideration your own life and family. Mama wouldn't want you to sacrifice for her anyway. She wants to be a blessing. If she lives far away, arrange to have someone check in on her, have groceries delivered, or whatever else she may need, and rest in that. If she chooses to move in with, or closer to you, then your responsibilities will change.

>>> **Your loved one may never have had to take care of their own mother or father.** Have you ever thought about that? And yet, you are doing the loving and responsible thing in caring for them. Again, give yourself some credit. You are doing the right thing, so go a little easier on yourself.

But what if, no matter what you do, Mama is miserable and unhappy?

In reality, there are some people who will never make the adjustment to their new life. If this is the case, you will probably find this has been the pattern of their life, and they like being unhappy. You may have to deal with a loved one who looks at the frozen yogurt sundae you snuck in for them, and all they can do is ask, "Where's the cherry?" Or they may tell you that the flowers you left work early to pick up, make their eyes water.

What do you do if they are just downright mean and cranky?

You make sure you don't let them manipulate you. That sounds like such a terrible term to use when addressing someone you love, but it does happen. Manipulation is a form of making someone do something that benefits the manipulator. It means to use shrewd or devious management for someone's own advantage. If your loved one is exhibiting some of this behavior, recognize it and deal with it.

Do what you can to bring joy to their life, and then go on with yours. Have you ever been around someone and felt yourself totally drained when you left? You're not feeling drained; you've been drained! We all carry energy in ourselves that can actually be measured. When you have visited with someone and you feel tired and weak when you leave, there has been an exchange of energy. Here's a clue, you were not the recipient of energy, you were the unsuspecting donor. Guard yourself against this happening.

You've heard the expression, "There are givers and takers in life," and that is never going to change. If you are dealing with a loved one who has been a taker all of their life, chances are they are not going to have a miraculous conversion at the end of their days. Since your loved one has already made their choice as to how they address life, you have liberty to make some choices of your own. Your heart desires to do the best you can for your loved one, but it can be awfully difficult to help someone find joy in life when they don't want to.

>>> **All you can do is continue being the best person you know how to be.** Don't try to make sense of how anyone can be so unappreciative. You do not have that nature, so you will blessedly never be able to understand it. Do all you can, so at the end of this journey, you will be able to look back and know you did the best you could under some very difficult circumstances. And finally, when you head for home after another one of those frustrating visits, let it go! Rest in the knowledge your loved one ultimately belongs to God.

<<< Crossroads >>>

Is there a community set up with hierarchies established, as they were in real life, and do you see the resident's personalities come forward?

Professional Caregiver's Response
Yes, only magnified! The divas come out. If they were outgoing in life, they are the ones organizing their little community. If they were loners, they will stay more to their rooms. If Mama didn't play bingo before, don't make her do it now.

Do residents try to make the family feel guilty, or in any way con their families?

Professional Caregiver's Response
They perk up and dress nicer and some do con and manipulate those that love them. Some try to make family members feel guilty. They will make family members jump through hoops, and the children need to reverse that manipulation.

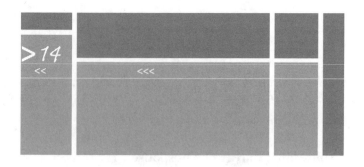

It's Not 30 Minutes—It's 30 Years!

Visiting Is Taking Its Emotional Toll

For where your treasure is, there will your heart be also.
—MATTHEW 6:21

YOUR DAILY, WEEKLY, OR MONTHLY VISIT DRAWS NEAR, and it is accompanied with apprehension, dread and fear. You hate that you are even having these feelings. You battle with your mind as you berate yourself for being selfish, unkind, and unfeeling. You're strung out like a tattered kite that is all out of wind. Tiredness has encompassed you and sometimes you wish it would all just end. Then guilt rears its ugly head, and the cycle begins again. You have to stop and think about this logically, because if you don't, you will crumble under the pressure.

But how can you be logical about this? You must assess your situation, realize the tremendous pressure you are under, and give yourself some grace. There is a way you can make those visits more enjoyable. Before you walk down those frosty corridors, kneel and bask in the warmth of the heavenly Father. The Lord can and will give you amazing strength to do this.

>>> **Build yourself up with prayer before you go visit your loved one.** You have made the visits so often that the unwanted scenario plays like a bad rerun in your mind. You pull into the parking lot and survey the other visitors as they scurry up the ramped entrance. Then it's your turn. You pull the door open, an odor assaults your nostrils, and you want to take flight. The attendants nod their heads as you walk down the florescent-lit hallways. The lights cast a yellowish cast on everyone's skin, and you can hear little moans, tired voices calling out from behind steel doors. Your heart is moved with helplessness, as you look at those who are slumped in wheelchairs, lined up like wooden soldiers. Some patients have gotten the hang of their new home and whisk by in their motorized freedom, sending a whiff of stale air past you.

What are they all waiting for, and how can you help them? Surprisingly, they are simply looking for a bright smile or a subtle touch. Your hands can transform their day. Reach out to them and watch their faces light up as their eyes take on a hint of recognition of a world bigger than their concrete cocoon. Do you see the change in them? That's all Mama wants. She knows how hard it is for you to see her like she is. Don't forget, you're not getting any younger either. You're noticing the receding hairline and the valleys of wrinkles on Mama, while she might just be seeing you all decked out in your Brownie uniform. Maybe she sees you floating down the aisle in your wedding dress or standing at attention as you received your diploma, or jogging down the field for a touchdown.

Everyone is time traveling on these visits. You escape in your mind to a time when Mama was culling beans on the front porch or planting pansies in her garden. Or maybe you see Dad teaching you to drive or tossing you a baseball. The small quarters your loved one is confined to almost make you nauseous as your eyes bounce around the tiny space. Memories of their comfortable home bombard you, and you begin the whole process of telling yourself it's not fair, this isn't what you wanted for them. The starched, military-folded sheets irk you as you think back on Mama's thick comforters mounded atop sheets that always smelled of sunshine and lavender. The steel bedside table with its two tiny drawers in no way resembles Mama's dainty lace-draped dresser where her precious Bible always laid.

Since Mama's eyesight has diminished, you wonder if she misses reading her Bible. The words that had always sustained and fed her are buried in a tiny drawer beside her bed she can't even open. Still, Mama always brightens when you appear and that also concerns you. Are you the only bright spot in her life? And if you are, then are you now responsible to be there 24/7 to keep her vital and alive?

Her tiny closet houses a few bathrobes and dressing gowns. You remember when she was so fussy about her clothing. Always the lady, everything had to be just perfect. You can't help but question what is going on in her mind. Does she miss all those things? To be honest, every time you visit Mama, you are, in fact, thinking of your own self, one day laying upon one of those rigid beds, staring blankly at the cream-colored walls. As hard as it may be, you can't allow yourself to go down those roads. It is very important that you stay in the moment and make it the best you can.

>>> **You need to understand that you don't have to do anything; Mama just loves to look at you.** She is surrounded by unfamiliar people and objects, but you bring "home" to her. In the totality of it all, people are really all there is in life. No matter how rich, smart, or energetic we are, all of our lives will be reduced to those we have loved and love us. Money doesn't dress up hospital walls, photos of loved ones do. Intelligence doesn't have answers for the fountain of youth, and vitality will one day wane.

Some loved ones may not hear, see, or be cognizant, but God will make a way for you to communicate with them when there seems to be no way. This is where modern medicine is set aside and the Great Physician takes over. Act on those quiet impressions you feel, no matter how subtle. Believe the Lord is directing you in how to meet the needs of the one who is desperately holding on to life.

Now, let's have a little humor here. Mama needs a good laugh. Remember humor is medicine for the body. But how can you be jovial when you know you have to leave Mama in this foreboding atmosphere and return to the comfort and security of your own family? Just give Mama 100 percent of yourself while you are there. Pour out of yourself into her, and then leave. Yes, just leave. You will be back, and you will once again bring a smile to Mama's face. Love and laugh with her, right where she is, because you *are* her world. Her spirit is not housed in the dimly lit room or the locked building, it's in her heart, and that has not gone anywhere.

Look at those 30 years whirling through your mind every time you visit Mama, as a blessing. You and Mama are time traveling, and the key is to both come together for a moment and embrace the time you are in. That collision of emotions will be enough to sustain you and Mama until the next visit. Now go home and relax. Frankly, Mama is probably tired of having you look at her with those sad eyes. She feels she is still here for a darn good reason, and from the looks of your face, it just might be you!

<<< Crossroads >>>

How do you deal with the guilt and loneliness of missing the loved one they used to be, when you were a child?

Family Caregivers' Responses

I purposely try not to think about how far he has deteriorated or how very incapable he is in his present condition, compared to how he was 10 or 20 years ago. It is very difficult to take. He ran a medical practice, performed surgery, and saved people's lives with his expertise/knowledge of medicine. I ask why. I feel it is unfair and wonder if it could have been prevented.

My mom was a great person to all her kids. I will miss her dearly, but I know a lot of her is in my soul. If I can be 10 percent of the father to my kids that my mom was to us, then I will know I was successful in life.

I try not to think about it because it makes me cry, and I don't have time for that. I miss just being able to enjoy Mom's company.

How do the residents prepare for family visits? Do they get excited or change their attitudes?

Professional Caregiver's Response
It depends on if the family lives out of town or not. The residents get very excited and surprisingly, sometimes their confusion actually disappears for a time. If the family lives away and previously only saw them two times a year, nothing has changed except the parent's address. Don't feel guilty.

<<<   >>>

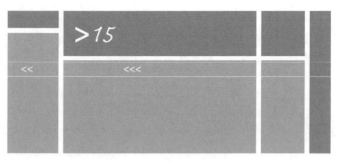

Changing of the Guard— You're the Captain Now

Keeping Family Traditions Now Rests in Your Hands

Therefore, brethren, stand fast, and hold the traditions which ye have been taught, whether by word, or our epistle.
—2 Thessalonians 2:15

TRADITIONS ARE THE FOUNDATION OF OUR LIVES. There is something very comforting in knowing that every year at Christmas Mama gives you a new set of dishtowels, and at Thanksgiving Dad always carves the turkey. At family gatherings, Dad always says grace, and Mama always calms the little ones down with her disapproving look.

In the back of your mind you have entertained thoughts, which you quickly suppressed, that there will come a day when things won't always be the same. As you watch your loved one grow frailer, each passing holiday brings the nagging anxiety they may not be around for the next one. It is a bitter, sweet emotion that brings a little fear with it.

Traditions are not only important to you, they are a stabilizing force in the lives of your children, who are used to going to Mama's every summer. Yes, they complain about it every year, but there is just something compelling about piling into the car at the crack of dawn with the expectations of Mama waiting on the porch, welcoming arms outstretched to greet them, and her warm apple tarts waiting in the kitchen. And Grandpa is the only one in the world that lets the boys mess around in his old tool shed.

>>> **Your children have memories of their own that bring stability to their lives.** They may buck and squawk as they are loaded into the car for another visit to Mama's, but once they get there, they enjoy the freedom they are given to roam and explore. They love having eager ears, waiting to hear every detail of their lives. Sometimes parents get very involved in everyday life, but kids know their grandparents are never too busy for them. Grandpa gets excited about the beetle bugs they catch, and Mama tucks them into bed under soft downy comforters.

>>> **The reason I am going into so much detail is so you remember there are other people involved in this whole process.** It is very easy to get caught up and believe you are the only one whose life will be affected by the loss of your loved one. Take some of your energy and use it to help others around you accept the situation. You will find yourself rising up in a strength and determination you didn't know you had. If you can replace your fear with faith, you will see the healing,

restorative power of the Lord in your life when you need it.

>>> **Though fear is a legitimate emotion in these circumstances, it does not have to dictate your behavior.** You don't know what your life will be like without the one you love and we are not creatures who are open to change—especially change that involves a huge gapping hole in our lives. For many, they are losing their confidant, their counselor, and their best friend. How does anyone prepare for something like that? How does anyone make the adjustment?

You accept the changes and ask the Lord how to make the most of the time you have with your loved one. Traditions are only brought forward if there is someone to carry the torch. Unfortunately, no matter how many siblings you have, there is usually only one who will step up to the plate and accept the responsibilities.

You are blessed if you are the one carrying the torch. I say blessed, because at the end of everything, you will discover amazing moments that others will not have experienced. It will be up to you to assemble extended family for holidays, see that Great Auntie Grace is picked up for Christmas, and send a special box of chocolates to Uncle Fred, just like Mama used to do.

I know it sounds like more work for you, but it's the little things you carry forward that will bring memories flooding back to others. Uncle Fred will be expectantly awaiting his box of chocolates, though in the back of his mind he knows Mama is not here anymore. The funny thing is, he doesn't even like chocolate. It was the fact that once a year he knew someone was thinking of him. Imagine his surprise when you send him a box of chocolates. Sweet memories will rush over him, memories of when he and Mama were kids, of how special she was to him and so many others.

You may never know the overflowing effects of your small gifts of kindness, but the Lord does. While you have this special time with your loved one, find out the history of your family's traditions. Gather all the information you can, and store it for the days to come. When it seems your world is being torn apart, your traditions are the glue that will piece it all back together again.

<<< Crossroads >>>

Are there any family traditions you sense might not be carried on—since your loved one is unable to enact them?

Family Caregiver's Response
I was always the driving force behind the family traditions. I loved Easter baskets and egg hunts. Thanksgiving dinners with all the trimmings, and Christmas. I struggled to continue these things after my loved one died, but the first year was heart-wrenching. It is me who is now unable to enact the traditions. Maybe I'll get back into the joyful habit, but it's been five years now, and I seem to have lost all desire for those things.

Do you worry that one day the things you enjoyed as a family with your loved one, will no longer be there?

Family Caregivers' Responses

I will miss my mom's ability to tell stories. She could find the humor and uniqueness in what others would see as ordinary moments, and she would convey them into something worthy of sharing.

>

I miss mom's ability to interact with others. We did volunteer work with handicapped children. She now needs consistency in her life, so she can be with us only for a couple of hours.

>

I love spending time with my mother. We shop and go dining and call each other every other day. One day, this will no longer be possible. I'll miss the time with her so much, but I'm so glad I am spending time with her now.

<<<   >>>

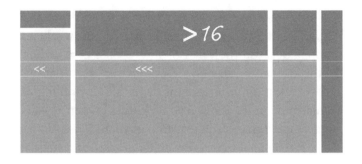

They Need New Shoes

Finances Are Stretched, Bank Accounts Diminished

Thou, O God, didst send a plentiful rain, whereby thou didst confirm thine inheritance, when it was weary.
—Psalm 68:9

Taking care of a loved one is an expensive, emotional roller coaster, and it does not ebb and flow with your work agenda or the kids' soccer schedule.

At work, you may find your mind is drifting when you should be concentrating on the spreadsheet in front of you. You wonder if Mama has taken her medication. Your leisurely lunch hours have been turned into shopping blasts for diapers and doctor updates, and your gourmet dinners have been replaced with fast foods.

Your concentration is not what it used to be at work, and people are noticing. You forgot the morning meeting because Mama had to have her tea, and you won't be able to attend the weekend seminar because there is no one to take care of her. All these changes may be affecting your job situation, and threatening your income, which is dwindling at an alarming rate. As everyone knows, when dollars get stretched, nerves get stretched with them.

>>> **You thought Mama was better prepared financially.** Surprise! Her insurance does not cover half of her medication. Nursing home costs have skyrocketed, and to get your loved one the care he or she needs, you are going to have to make some major adjustments in your own lifestyle.

The job promotion you were working toward will have to wait for another time because you know in your heart that you can't honestly give 100 percent of yourself. The new car your family was going to purchase smiles at you every time you drive by the car lot, and your children's college fund has not had a deposit made in it for six months. There are so many little bumps in the road that you didn't plan for. But in reality, how could you? You have essentially acquired another household to support and manage. Whew! Take a moment and congratulate yourself. Look around. Are there any other family members who have offered to help? Probably not. You have taken on a huge responsibility that comes with big sacrifices and even bigger heartaches.

This is where some bitterness can take root if your faith is not firmly entrenched in the Lord. The job you have taken on is one that doesn't offer any pay raises, promotions, or awards. There will be few onlookers cheering you on and no adulation from any co-workers.

No one will admire the ease with which you juggle two households, and there will be no words of praise for your administrative skills. In fact, the only one who will ever know what this has cost you, is the Lord.

Your nine-to-five job has enlarged to being on call 24 hours a day, and your pay has been cut in half. All of these changes are going to affect your life. You will feel guilty about not pulling your weight at work, guilty about being too tired to go to your kid's soccer game, and guilty about slighting your spouse. So what can you do about all the guilt you are feeling?

Refuse to let guilt become the motivating force in your life. Guilt never comes alone, it brings with it feelings of inadequacy, failure, depression, and sadness. It constantly tells you there is more you should or could do. Guilt is a hungry enemy that will slowly eat away at you unless you recognize it for what it is and stand against it with the Word of God. Get a Scripture you can pull out of your arsenal to stand against the wiles of the enemy. You can't logically outthink guilt, you have to supersede its power with a higher one. Here's where the Scriptures come in:

> *"Finally, brethren, whatsoever things are true, whatsoever things are honest, whatsoever things are just, whatsoever things are pure, whatsoever things are lovely, whatsoever things are of good report; if there be any virtue, and if there be any praise, think on these things"* (Philippians 4:8).
>
> or
>
> *"Therefore there is no condemnation to those who are in Christ Jesus"* (Romans 8:1).

The Word of God is the only power you have that can override your negative thinking. Why? Because the Word is designed to make you an overcomer, in any situation you are in. Even Jesus, when face-to-face with Satan, only used the Word. He didn't argue His case or listen to what others had to say about Him. He fully depended on the fact God loved Him and had empowered Him with an invaluable tool, the Word.

>>> **Open your Bible and see what He is telling you about your situation.** Find out what His expectations for you are. He is a loving Father who knows exactly where you are. He sees you struggling to pay your bills, and He knows you would do anything in your power to help the one you love. It's just that sometimes, things are taken out of our control. When they are, at that point, just let them go.

You may be saying, "That's easy for you to say; you don't know or understand the situation I am in." Granted, I don't, but God does and He told us to come to Him, all who are weary and heavy laden, and He will give us rest (See Matthew 11:28.). If we believe, then here's where we have to let things go.

Mama is not looking for you to put her up in a five-star hotel or provide her every whim; she just wants to be near you. Don't forget the whole purpose of our existence— to love. You can't work yourself into proving that you love Mama, she knows you do. Just like you know she loved you when you were spattered in mud, failing in school, and driving her crazy with your teenage late hours.

If you are honest with yourself, a lot of the work you are doing, is to keep that old guilt at bay. Become the master of guilt, and you will find you are freer to enjoy being with Mama. A hug is more substantial than a square meal, a touch is more valuable than a fancy bathrobe, and a kiss is more significant than whatever you are drumming up in your mind that you should have done.

>>> **Your finances will recover over time, but your heart won't if you don't take some time to invest in what is really important.** If you look at your present state as just that, present, then you can look past where you are today. This is just a momentary blip in your life that will eventually end. Your world will resume its normalcy. It will be in those days that you will understand and actually yearn for the days when you had to interrupt your work to make Mama a cup of tea. But in the meantime, try to enjoy that shoestring budget, because you're tied up with the one you love!

<<< Crossroads >>>

How are you handling the additional financial stress associated with caring for your loved one?

Family Caregivers' Responses

Currently well. However, when this adventure began, we had no idea where the money would come from. Thanks to God, a good elder-lawyer, a small inheritance given to my mother and Medicaid, things look much better.

>

My mom lives with my brother so at this time I am not responsible for any finances. However, there could come a time when I will have to help. Depending on how long my mom lives, I might be affected.

>

Over the three years my loved one was dying, I went from "struggling" to "flat out broke and about to lose my house." I was so busy working two jobs and coming home to feed, bath, and take care of him, that I neglected to take care of the finances like I should have. Soon I was at rock bottom and the bank had filed for foreclosure before I finally faced facts and got my act together. The strength to do all that came directly from God. He led me, step by step, from chaos to victory.

How has caring for your loved one affected your job performance, advancement, and career goals?

Family Caregivers' Responses

In the beginning it was rough because my mother lived with us and I was very distracted. Now that she is in an assisted living facility, the only time I miss from work is to take her to doctor appointments.

>

My heart wasn't in my job, so my performance was bare minimum, and sometimes slipped below that. I was easily frustrated and burst into tears at inappropriate times, or lost my temper when I shouldn't have. I was also a very private person, so most of my co-workers and supervisors had no idea what was causing my high absenteeism or mood swings. I wanted so desperately to change jobs - to find a new career (to run away). I knew that when my loved one died, I would be able to make any and all the changes I wanted to. And I did.

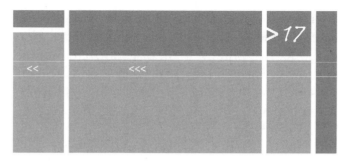

Bacon and Biscuits Beckon You Home

Sometimes Memories Are All You Have; They're Enough

Let them be before the LORD continually, that he may cut off the memory of them from the earth.
—PSALM 109:15

MEMORIES ARE A VERY POWERFUL FORCE. THEY'RE A vital component of who you are today, and they affect a lot of the decisions you will make tomorrow. Good memories can take you to a restful place, and bad memories can haunt you.

Many people are dealing with elderly loved ones who no longer recognize them, and only the power of God and His grace can help them through the trying days. Some people have loved ones who can no longer communicate with them, while others are caring for a parent with dementia who is frightened to be around their own children.

How do you deal with all of these changes? You have to either go back in your mind to those great memories that bring you joy, or go forward into the unknown, which brings anxiety. It sounds so cut-and-dried, but in reality, what choice do you have?

And think of Mama; put yourself in her place. Would you want your children worrying about you or would you rather they think about all the good times you had? Memories are a validation that Mama did something right. It's the gentle memories that will carry you through the tough days.

You remember how Mama used to save the ends of a loaf of bread to feed the birds, or how she used to drive you crazy organizing the silverware drawer. The memories of your loved one actually define how you saw that person. They are the details in your loved one's life that made an impact on you.

>>> **Like small diamonds in the darkness, memories light up your past life and bring you a gentle respite from the harshness of reality.** When the bills are mounting, the doctors want you to make yet another decision, and you're so tired you can't even eat, then is the time to close your eyes and remember when life seemed a little easier and a whole lot safer. After all, Mama was in charge, and her strength never seemed to diminish. She always had the answers you needed, even in times when she never said a word.

What's important to your loved one is that you remember.

Not everyone had perfect parents. In fact, no parent is perfect, but that is life. If you missed out on a blissful childhood, it may be a little harder to recall those memories, but they are there. You may have to scale your expectations down a little, but it will be worth it. Don't look for fireworks and crystal moments, look for moments when you felt safe and happy. The media has dramatized life. In reality, life is not huge shopping sprees or front-row concert seats; it's moments of wonder and learning. That's what your loved one did for you.

They took the time to teach you how to tie your shoes, button your shirt, and put one and one together to make two. Somehow you have been transformed from a helpless baby to a successful adult, and there are a whole lot of memories along the way. Your loved one was instrumental in getting you where you are today. Instead of looking for flaws, consider the sacrifices made for you. Mama passed up opportunities in her life because you had needs. She laid down her own dreams in order to lift you up, and she had her own expectations that were never met because you were more important to her. So travel back again in your mind with a different point of view. You will find some amazing moments you missed along the way.

>>> **And what will your own children think and remember about you?** Believe me, it won't be those $100 sneakers you did or didn't buy for them. It will be the time you put your work aside and helped them catch fireflies or bake cookies. The exciting thing about life is that you have the ability to choreograph a great part of it. You decide what you are going to do, and today, you can create special memories for your loved ones.

As long as Mama is here, there is still time for making memories. They are created in the mishaps of life, the small gestures of kindness, and the words of love that you speak. You may be disappointed that Mama is not fulfilling the memories you have of her baking flaky biscuits or frying bacon, but that doesn't mean you can't create new ones today.

>>> **Take her outside and watch a sunrise together.** Bundle her up and let her feel the cold air as you both sip hot chocolate. If she can't go outside, bring out the old photo albums and the two of you snuggle up. Put on an old black-and-white movie as you brush her hair or put lotion on her hands.

It's the smile you are looking for. The look in her eyes, assuring you she feels safe, is what you will remember. So put aside all of your worries for a short time, and direct your energies to making some lasting memories. Mama just wants to know you are there for her, and all of your wisdom and skills fall short compared to a simple cup of hot chocolate.

And yes, sometimes life really is just that simple.

<<< Crossroads >>>

What lasting memory would you like your loved one to have of your attempts to give them the best life you possibly could?

Family Caregivers' Responses

To know that I was always there for him...that he could always count on me when needed. And know that I tried to comfort him, as best I could.

>

As my mom gave her time to me when I was a baby, I, in turn, am giving her my time in her time of need.

>

That we tried our best, and we loved her with all of our hearts.

<<<   >>>

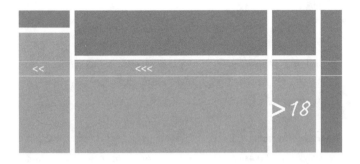

Where's the Instruction Manual?

Decisions—You Are Holding Someone's Life in Your Hands

But let him ask in faith, nothing wavering. For he that wavereth is like a wave of the sea driven with the wind and tossed.
—JAMES 1:6

DECISIONS, DECISIONS, DECISIONS. SUDDENLY strangers in white coats and cold steely eyes are looking expectantly at you, as they tap the metal binder that holds your loved one's medical history. Mama's warm, giving heart has been reduced to beats per minute, and her tired eyes are referred to as dilated pupils. The slow gentle nodding of her head is written up as sluggish motor reflexes, and her diminished appetite is depicted as someone who needs a feeding tube.

It is very difficult for children to watch their parents fade from once vigorous human beings, to weak, dependent patients, but it is inevitable. We are all losing our grip on youth. Think of yourself. I'm sure there is something you can find that you could do years ago, but can't do today. To come to terms with what is occurring in your loved one's life you need to lean on Jesus. He is the author and finisher of your faith, and He sees how hard it is for you to cope with the situation.

>>> **I wish there was a ten-step program I could direct you to that would merrily carry you through the journey you are on, but there is none.** You are going to be faced with a lot of decisions to make over the next couple of months, or years. Decisions that are difficult to make.

Who can make the decision to turn off a respirator that is keeping a loved one alive? Who can make the decision to send Mama to surgery or not? We don't know ahead of time the outcome of the choices we make. Nor are we given any guarantees or warranties from the medical arena. If you make a mistake, there is no going back.

And how are you expected to know what Mama wants? Even though she might have left a living will, there is still a lot of individual interpretation as to what it says. Mama said she did not want to be kept alive with artificial means, but the doctors tell you that if they don't put a feeding tube in, she will never regain her strength to get well. Mama never wanted to be resuscitated, but she only coded because the medication was the wrong dose.

So how do you know when you have gone past Mama's will, or the Lord's? Technically, if you took the machinery off of any seriously ill patient, the patient would expire; but in many cases, some people only need a little help mechanical to get over what is ailing them. However, there are cases where the machinery is the only thing keeping someone alive.

Since you are not a medical doctor, how are you to make these huge decisions? Where is the manual of life, telling you step-by-step how to assemble or disassemble someone's life? We don't have a problem index or troubleshooter, like we have with our computers or electronic gadgets, to tell us if our loved one is doing this, then we should do this. How do you collect the information you need to make the right decisions?

>>> **Communication. If you haven't done so already, sit down and have a healthy, open discussion with your loved one.** They are not afraid to talk about it—you are. They know you are uneasy with the task at hand, but you might be surprised how open they are to discuss something that is so important to them.

When they talk about what they do or don't want, have them be specific. You won't be able to get an answer for every scenario, but you will get the intent of their heart. If you listen past their words, you can get a sense of where they are coming from and what they are thinking. Remember, this is their life, and they do have the right to define the integrity of it.

You might be in a place where your loved one is unresponsive. Here is where you need to evaluate the person they once were and the quality of life they would, or would not, be satisfied living. Don't make the mistake of thinking *if it were me*. You may have an entirely different personality than your loved one. You could be an energetic, world traveler, whereas your loved one has always been content to just sit in a chair and watch the squirrels play in the yard.

If you keep your loved one's interest in the middle of your decision making, then you can be assured your motives are pure. This is important, so that in the days to come questions don't overwhelm you.

Once Mama tells you what she considers a quality life, then promise her you will carry out her wishes. She is depending on you to act on her behalf when she can no longer do it. At that point in her life, she is not expecting you to second-guess or circumvent her desires just because you want her with you. She is not leaving decisions in your hands, she is leaving the carrying out of her decisions to you, and that's a big difference.

>>> **If you get into turmoil, open the best manual available: the Bible.** It has all the answers you need. God has a way of getting answers to His children that we cannot explain. You may have read a passage fifty times, but when you needed an answer, it spoke to you. Go figure! Why did it speak to your heart this time and not the other times you read it? Could it be previously you were dull of hearing? Or maybe you were too busy to let the spirit of the Lord minister to you. Could it have been you read the passage, but your mind was on your grocery list? No one knows the answers to any of the above, and it doesn't really matter anyway. What matters is you needed direction from Him, and He spoke to you through His Word.

Over the ensuing days, rejoice that you are not alone, nor are you the sole one making decisions. Your loved one has probably already had an audience with the Lord, and He knows exactly what they requested. He will honor the promises He made to them, and you are the blessed one called to enact those promises.

The Lord has provided you a manual of life that is 1,189 chapters long and filled with expert advice, wisdom, and guidance. So the next time you find yourself in a dilemma, get your Bible out, let your fingers do the walking though the Scriptures, and let the Spirit of the Lord do the talking.

<<< Crossroads >>>

Have you had a talk with your loved one about the extent of care they want and do they have a living will?

Family Caregivers' Responses
Yes, mom has made it clear for years that she doesn't want any "heroic" health care.

>

I don't know what my mom wants.

Do you think you will be able to abide by your loved one's wishes without feeling guilty?

Family Caregivers' Responses
I believe so since these are her wishes and I believe she will go to heaven. However, I think at the time I will have an internal conflict between wanting to do all I can to help her while still abiding by her wishes.

>

I hope and pray the Lord will give me the strength to be there with my husband to help him make the decisions for his mother.

Have you had to make any major medical decisions on behalf of your loved one?

Family Caregiver's Response
My brother and I had to decide to withhold care from my mother recently, but she made a comeback. It was difficult at the moment but we realized it was our mother's wishes.

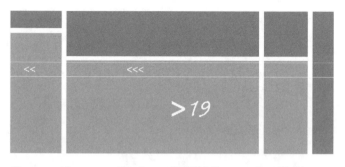

Superhero, Take Off Your Cape— Put On Your Garment of Praise

Juggling Two Households? You Need Another Hand

To appoint unto them that mourn in Zion, to give unto them beauty for ashes, the oil of joy for mourning, the garment of praise for the spirit of heaviness; that they might be called trees of righteousness, the planting of the Lord, that he might be glorified.
—Isaiah 61:3

YOU COME STRAGGLING IN THE DOOR FROM WORK AND immediately get overwhelmed. There sits a cold stove, the kids' homework to check, and a mound of bills to be paid. After working all day, you now have to overcome the guilt as you pop a frozen meal into the microwave and hastily glance over the kids' paperwork. Your mind wanders back to a time when you used to anticipate leisurely chopping up a crisp salad, as sweet onions sizzled in the frying pan. The whole evening used to stretch out before you with so many choices. Should you have a nice cup of coffee and curl up with a book, or should you prop up for the night with a bowl of popcorn and a good movie?

>>> **Trying to figure out how your life got so disjointed is a futile waste of precious energy.** Your life today is what it is, and to try and make it anything else will bring you frustration, and maybe even some anger. Great minds today attempt to drill into our heads that we should live in the moment. That is great advice, unless you desperately want the moment to end and a better one to begin. How are you supposed to ignore the tremendous pressure you feel? And until someone comes up with a new financial exchange that turns the value of dollar bills into thousands, you must deal with your diminishing finances.

You are exhausted, and that's OK. Your physical body can take only so much, and you are now experiencing burn out. And how about your mind, which is zipping faster than a computer deleting files as it crashes? Your monthly visits to the hairdresser and manicurist have been replaced with Mama's doctor appointments, and you have depleted all of your sick days at work. Is there any respite coming? How long do you think you can go on at your present pace?

>>> **You are not alone in asking these questions.** Others dealing with similar circumstances may appear to be doing just fine, but don't let their smiling faces fool you. As humans, we are unique, but in dealing with situations, there is really very little difference in the way we react to unwanted changes in our lives. It's time you started to pat yourself on the back a little more and give yourself some mercy. If you are waiting for the other members of your family—who

have silently looked away from the situation—to stand up and applaud your heroic attempt at taking care of Mama, you will be disappointed. People are people, and as stated before, some are givers and some are takers. You're the giver, and the takers are relieved someone else is handling the situation, even though they should be doing their fair share. Here is where another old saying comes in—"out of sight, out of mind."

It doesn't do any good to get angry with other family members for not helping, because you are not going to change one little thing, except increase your consumption of aspirin and antacids. Reading this, it might seem you are in a no-win situation. But the one thing Christians have is hope that pops up and propels us forward. As long as we have hope, the blueprint of faith, we can find the strength and fortitude we need from the Lord.

To activate hope, you must make your mind and body do things they don't want to do. How do you tell your exhausted body that it is now going to raise its tired arms and praise the Lord? And how can you look over your cluttered house and thank the Lord for another day to dust and mop the floors?

And why should you do any of the above anyway? Doesn't the Lord see you need help? Where is He and why has He not fixed the situation? Why, why, why?

It's as if you are in a box with the lid sealed shut, and there is no way out. You feel helpless and alone because you can't change, fix, or alter anything. And forget about the Lord opening a door when He closes another. You can't even see a sliver of light from under the locked door in front of you. What is a body to do?

Venting is good, and that is what we have just done in the above paragraphs. It allows thoughts that you have been trying to suppress to come tumbling out into the open. Call it a mental purge. You've just hit the defrag button of your mind, and all of those negative, random thoughts are being collected into one sector before they are deleted. So your venting is really the beginning of a necessary process your brain needs to go through to enable it to move forward.

>>> **Another way to move on is to acknowledge that you can't do it all, and you surely can't continue at the level of excellence you have been requiring of yourself.** Back down those high expectations and release some pressure on yourself. We've talked a lot about Mama in this book, but unless you get yourself under control, you can't help anyone. There is nothing wrong, and everything right, with focusing a little on your own needs. Recognize there are a lot of demands being put on you and devise a few options to free yourself from the burdens. It is amazing what ten minutes of solitude can do.

>>> **Go outside and watch the sunset; dinner can wait.** Put on the garment of praise and thanksgiving. Unless you get very still inside, you won't be able to see the glorious painted sky or hear the chirping crickets. God's creation is magnificent and can only be experienced if you take the time. You are not going to see His glory if you are racing around the house collecting the laundry or checking your email. It takes effort to slow down, recenter, and realign yourself with His will.

When you breathe the fresh air and listen to His creatures preparing for nightfall, it thrusts you into another dimension. You begin to reconnect with His restorative powers. You might not be able to praise Him for the workload awaiting you, but you can honestly praise Him for the wonderful world He created for your enjoyment. Praise Him for the cool breeze brushing your cheek, the gently swaying of the maple tree, the myriad of colors painting the sky, and the blessing of having one more day to walk among His creation with the ones you love.

Sometimes it is very difficult to clear your mind and get started, but once you do, the spirit of the Lord inside of you will awaken. It is His Spirit that picks you up off your bed every morning and hovers over you as you sleep. Man's power has limitations, and when we are weak, He is strong. If you feel you have reached the end of your own ability and really can't go on one more day unless something changes, now is the time to reach into the spiritual realm where God lives.

Ten minutes can make all the difference in how you handle the next few hours with your family. They are not really concerned about how fresh or nutritious the salad is, they just want to see you happy and listening to what they have to say.

Your time giving praise and thanksgiving to the Lord may not have changed your situation, but it did change one thing…you!

<<< Crossroads >>>

Do you have siblings, and are they participating in the care of your loved one? If they are not, how do you feel and deal with that?

Family Home Caregivers' Responses

Many people do feel resentment that other siblings may not devote enough time for the caring of loved ones. I do have a brother and sister, but I do not feel any anger, irritation, or frustration that they do not help as much as I do. Initially, I did harbor some of these feelings, but I no longer feel that way.

I have sisters, and they have been very little help in this process. I realize some people can step up and contribute, and others are emotionally unable to. I hold no ill feelings, and I know God gives me daily strength.

<<< >>>

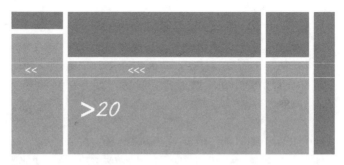

They've Changed, But So Have You!

Did You Ever Think You Had It in Yourself?

When I was a child, I spake as a child, I understood as a child, I thought as a child: but when I became a man, I put away childish things.
—1 Corinthians 13:11

THROUGH THIS JOURNEY WITH YOUR LOVED ONE, YOU are experiencing a lot of ups and downs, and it seems there are a whole lot more downs than ups. Watching the decline of someone we love is difficult. You will not escape unscathed from this experience, but you may be surprised at what you have learned along the way. Life is like one huge textbook that some people immerse themselves in and learn from while others merely scan over it.

You have done things you never thought you could and made decisions you never knew you had the wisdom to do. You've been scared by emotions that have surfaced and, at the same time, experienced moments of miraculous peace.

Some people feel great contentment with the situation, while others rage in their souls. You may have faithfully prayed every day and not seen any miraculous change. This tends to make the winds of your soul turn into Category 5 hurricanes, and there is no way to calm down. Your frustration level has shot to a dangerous level, and woe be unto the person who takes your parking place. You've lost all hope and feel like an empty shell inside. Thoughts are running through your head telling you it doesn't matter if you pray or not because no one hears you. Your prayers are just words spoken into the wind.

Then you begin to doubt everything you've ever read in the Bible, leaving you with nowhere to go with your questions. You feel like a trapped rat as you watch Mama deteriorate. You've done all you know to do, and others tell you it will be OK, but right about now, you feel nothing will ever be OK again. Your mind reprimands you that you should have more faith, because Mama is depending on you to fix the situation.

>>> **If you have gone through any of this, questioned your relationship with your Father, or doubted His faithfulness, you are not alone.** It is natural when we are in difficult situations to reach out to a higher power and hopefully expect something to change. It's how you handle the disappointment that will change you. Disappointment can either make your faith a whole lot stronger, or it will crush it. Either way, it is going to require you to trust in the Lord and hold steady.

If your faith drains out of your feet every time you see Mama, you may be shaken for a while, but you will be OK. Your tiny seed of faith will never leave you, and it will be the small sliver of light that the Lord will use to brighten your world once again.

Those who are content with the situation will find they have changed also, because their faith brought them the reassurance they needed, to hold fast to what they believed in. It's that brick upon brick theory. Layer upon layer of faith and trust have accomplished what they needed to do—to build a wall of protection around their heart. This is not to say one person is farther ahead spiritually than the other. It just means everyone is at a different place in their relationship with the Lord. Some may believe the Lord for miracles and think nothing is impossible to him who believes, while others accept what is as the Lord's will.

There are people who have questions. They've howled at the moon, raised their fists to the heavens, and wanted to know why. Mama was kind to everyone, and she now has been abused by the system. She never hurt a soul in her life, and now she lies on her bed in such pain. She gave when she had nothing to give, and now when she needs something, there is nothing. She helped so many people, now where is the help for her?

>>> **Watching a loved one slowly decline will change anyone.** You may develop deep scars that will take a long time to heal, and you may feel relief that Mama is finally going home to her reward. Resign yourself to the fact there is great change coming to your life, and all you can do is love your loved one. Realize

there will be good and bad days. Seize the good ones, and pray away the bad ones.

Either way, you will be changed. But there is one thing that never changes, and that is, when you are ready, your Father will still be waiting to comfort you.

<<< Crossroads >>>

What troubles you the most?

Family Caregivers' Responses

To see him in his current state of incapability, both physically and mentally, is extremely troubling. Presently, he still recognizes me, but I know in time he will reach a point where he doesn't.

>

I will miss her so much when that day comes. If God would give me one wish, it would be to turn the clock back..

<<<   >>>

It's Time to Take Them for a Walk

The Signs Are All There—
Don't Miss Your Opportunities

So likewise ye, when ye shall see all these things, know that it is near, even at the doors.
—MATTHEW 24:33

THERE ARE HUNDREDS OF SIGNS ALL AROUND YOU: Mama doesn't speak like she used to, her frail hand can't hold a cup, and she can barely nod her head. You can walk around in denial ignoring all of the signs, or you can reassure Mama you are there for her. Talk to her about your anxiety, and invite her to tell you what she is feeling. You don't want one precious minute to pass in subterfuge.

To experience the richness in life, you must consciously enter moments and go to the depths of where they lead you, or you will never see the glorious heights to which these moments can take you. These moments are the reality of life, and they're not sugar-coated with Mama beautifully coifed, sitting up in bed. In fact, she will probably be lying under harsh florescent lights and wearing a faded hospital gown.

>>> **Now is the time to dig deep and truly discover what the person you love is made of.** Ask Mama questions about things that have bothered you for years. The demons that have haunted you from your childhood can be chased away with a simple explanation from her. Ask her about all those subjects that were taboo for the family to discuss. Air out that dirty laundry!

Almost all families have those hush-hush things no one talks about but everyone has heard tidbits of. Dive right in there. Encourage Mama to open up. Many people have been carrying secrets for years, and it is liberating to tell someone about them. You might be surprised to learn Aunt Lisa was a diva or Grandpa had a secret desire for car racing. It's exciting to learn of your history, and it gives you a more complete picture of your loved one. We forget they were once young, daring, in love, and had extraordinary visions for their own lives. Let Mama fill in some of those blanks in both your lives.

Don't leave any room for regrets that can worry you the rest of your life. Regrets have a way of popping up at the most importune times, bringing depression and self-condemnation with them. If you have anything at all you would love to do, or say to your loved one, now is the time for it. Let your guard down, and allow yourself to get a little crazy. Right now you have the opportunity to make some of the most memorable moments you will ever have.

Let propriety fall by the wayside! Bundle Mama up, and drive her to the park for a picnic. At the hospital or nursing home, bring in some dainty china, a delicate tablecloth, and some delicious tea. Ignore all of the negative thoughts bombarding you. You know, the ones telling you it isn't seemly, there are too many medical issues to deal with, and how in the world are you going to get the facility to allow you to do such a thing. Forget about all of those things and go for it!

Special moments are created, they don't just spontaneously occur. To make them happen, you must be courageous and totally focused on what's best for your loved one. Is it really better they sit in a wheelchair and stare glumly out of the window, or would you prefer them to hear the invigorating noise of the city, feel the cool wind on their face, see a bumblebee, or touch the fresh grass? Sometimes you have to override what the sensible thing to do is, and let your emotions dictate the path you take.

Your loved one has invested a huge part of their heart and life into you, and that is a phenomenal gift. Take this time to open up your soul to the one you love. Their first concern is probably you, not themselves. They are afraid you won't be able to take care of yourself. They are concerned that once they are gone, you won't be able to handle their leaving, and worried they might not have done all they needed to do to prepare you for their leaving.

>>> **Every day you spend with your loved one is a beautifully wrapped gift.** You have the ability to open that package and enjoy all the wonders of life, or you can choose to never undo the ribbon and always wonder what could have been.

It is all up to you how the last days with your loved one will be. There will be circumstances you have no control over, but for the most part, you alone are the one who will dictate how you are going to react to a situation. You can sit on the sidelines and watch your loved one's passage into a new life, or you can walk side by side with them until they enter another dimension. The Lord will give you the strength you need to pass your loved one's life into His capable hands. Remember, Mama belongs to Him; she was only on loan to you.

Help Mama walk with grace into the outstretched arms of Her savior and when she looks back, let her see you, her baby, smiling as she goes.

<<< Crossroads >>>

What will you remember most about this journey you have been on?

Family Caregivers' Responses

My mom never wanted to be placed in a nursing home and did not like doctors. I know her wish has been granted, and I am glad I was here to help fulfill it. This time I'm spending with her is priceless, time that I will never forget.

>

The simple fact that he still recognizes me when I see him, he smiles and says my name, he is still with me, so I can spend time with him. These are different pleasures than I used to have, but these are now the pleasures I feel and cherish.

>

I am aware of what the next phases of the disease will entail. I do not think that I will ever fully be able to accept this or be prepared for it. I am afraid of what lies ahead for my father and the care he will need.

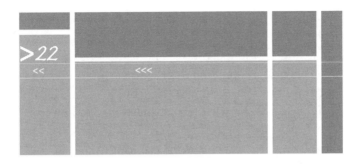

Reaffirm, Reassure, and Release

It's Now or Never

When the perishable has been clothed with the imperishable, and the mortal with immortality, then the saying that is written will come true: "Death has been swallowed up in victory."
—1 Corinthians 15:54

This journey you are on has no detours. There was a beginning, and there will be an end. Mama was there when you took your first step, and she watched you experience the joys of life. She saw your glee as you cuddled a puppy, heard your laughter as you chased a butterfly, and tasted your tears as she held you close when the world turned upside down on you. Now it's your turn.

As she watched you take your first wobbly step into life, then you, rightly so, will watch her take her first step out of life. Just as she was there for you, you need to be there for her. She couldn't promise you a perfect life, but she let you know that no matter what, she would be there. The same goes for you. You can't guarantee her what is to come in the afterlife, only the Word can do that, but you can let her know you will be with her as she steps into eternity. The Lord has a place prepared for all of us, and for those who believe, His Word is enough.

>>> **Now is the time to reassure Mama that you will be OK.** Let her know how much she means to you, and comfort her in her time of loss. Remember she is losing everyone she loves. Give her a sense of peace, so she can go on to her reward with the Lord. Your loved one has left a lot behind already. They've released their home, their possessions, and what used to be. Everything falls to the wayside when you are looking at months, days, or hours. They are destiny driven, and desperately holding on to love, which is the most valuable thing there is.

You can help ease their anxiety and fear by just being there with them. Hold their hand, rub their brow, and see that they are getting the best possible care available. Feed their souls by reading the Bible to them and leave music playing when you are not there. Even if they are not cognizant, their soul still is.

You are going to need a lot of help from the Lord at this time, and the only place you can get it, is on your knees. There are no short cuts or bullet points to get you through this one. You have important things to do, so lay all of your questions, anger, and frustrations at His feet. You need to be full of hope and clear minded. Mama wants to be reassured that you will to be able to go on without her, so don't disappoint her.

Sitting there weeping at her bedside does not mean you love her any more than if you chat cozily beside her bed. What would you want to remember about your own children? What kind of behavior would bring you the greatest peace?

>>> **Spend all the time you can with Mama, give her 100 percent of the best you have, and then you can collapse into the arms of Jesus.** But while you are with your loved one, ask the Lord to give you the strength to do things you don't want to do and the courage to let your loved one go. Keep Mama's needs paramount in your mind, and you will find amazing perseverance to be the strong individual she knows you to be.

If you can change your thinking from the panic mode of "She may be gone within the next few minutes or hours," to a serene, "I am blessed to have each minute," then you will utilize every second with your loved one. Everyone loses people they love, and it wounds to the core, no matter who it is. The goal is to remember this is about Mama. It's about what is best for her, what she wants and how she chooses to leave this life.

You've seen that her property was dealt with, as she requested. You've handled all of the medical and legal affairs that she entrusted to you. Now, you need to give the reins back to Mama. She's the one in charge here. Her body is preparing itself to make that miraculous change from mortality to immortality, and there is no going back. She may have already had a taste of the glory to come, and she's got one foot on earth and one in heaven. Her heart is telling her to stay for you, and her Lord is beckoning her to come home, with Him. She yearns to see her grandchildren grow up, and yet Jesus has assured her they will be OK without her.

What a dilemma! And you thought you were the one so confused. Stand back for just a second and look at the situation from Mama's perspective. She would be the first one to tell you she had a good life, and her stay on earth was to accomplish all He had given her to do. When Mama looks at you, she knows she has completed the most important job He gave her, which was to raise you up in the way you should go. You are Mama's greatest accomplishment, and her finest hours were those she spent with you.

Celebrate her life with smiles of endearment, hugs of thankfulness, and tears of gratitude, and then let her make the final decision. She let you run the show for a while, but Mama will be center stage, taking the final bow all by herself! Stand up and give her an ovation for the phenomenal life she lived.

<<< Crossroads >>>

What changes, if any, would you make?

Family Caregiver's Response
My father has always been one to do anything for me when I was a kid. Now I see this as my way of doing the same for him, repaying him for what he has done for me. He was always there for me to lend support, and I want to ensure that I can say I did the same for him.

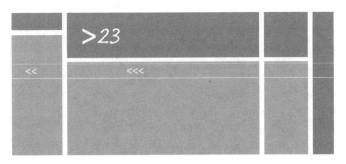

Your Mortality Immersed in a Baptism of Fire

They're Gone and You Are No One's Child

He answered and said, Lo, I see four men loose, walking in the midst of the fire, and they have no hurt; and the form of the fourth is like the Son of God.
—DANIEL 3:25

MAMA IS GONE AND YOUR LIFE FEELS SO EMPTY. How could her very existence have been reduced to that one little blue suitcase you took from the hospital? You stand under the old oak tree clutching what is left of Mama's life, and you hear the birds singing. The sky is a brilliant sapphire, dotted with wispy white clouds, and you smell newly mowed grass. It is a surreal moment. It's as if no one knows Mama is gone. How can the world just keep going on, as if nothing monumental has occurred? Doesn't anyone realize she is gone?

As you unpack the suitcase, you still smell her scent on the clothes. You wash and neatly pack them away. Her hairbrush still holds a few gray wisps of hair and her dog-eared Bible displays her handwriting where she made little notes in the margins. Her scruffy slippers remind you of how she used to shuffle along the hallway, and her worn change purse makes you smile. She used to be so diligent with the little money she had.

You think about all of the boxes you've got stored in the garage that need to be gone through. You can't do that just yet. How can you look at Mama's glasses and not see them perched on her tiny nose? How can you hold Dad's hunting jacket, knowing he will never amble through the woods again? And how can you seal those boxes with masking tape? You feel like you are packing up their life and disposing of it. It may be a necessary thing to do, but it's so final. You hate doing it and think about putting it off. Those boxes represent places you are not ready to go yet. They contain too many memories that will turn your heart inside out.

Just when you thought the hard part was over, here comes another hurdle. By now, you are tired of jumping and being sideswiped by another emotional blast. This journey has taken you on roads you never knew existed, and you've gotten lost in the woods a few times. There have been so many detours that you are dizzy, and the Lord's navigational system you've been depending on has you wondering if He realizes you are lost.

You can't stop crying, and you want to pummel someone, or something, to get out the anger you feel. Is it anger or is it a huge yearning inside of yourself that you know will never be filled again? And there is tremendous frustration because this is something you can't fix or change. There is no going back, and right now, it seems, there is no going forward. How can you handle the fact that you will never see your loved one again until you yourself enter heaven?

And how do you know she is OK? You look for some kind of sign that she made it to the other side. You try to make a deal with the Lord that if He will just let you see her one more time, everything will be OK. But you know in your heart of hearts that if you saw Mama one more time it wouldn't be enough.

>>> **No one can prepare themselves for the loss of a loved one, but blessedly you have the Lord.** He is the Comforter, and though it seems there is no comforting for you right now, when you look back months from now, you will see Him. You will see His presence in the smile Mama had on her face when she left you. His shoulder is what you leaned on when you couldn't stand up, and His arm is what encompassed you when the pain of losing Mama got so bad.

And all those doubts you keep having as to whether your loved one really knew how much you loved them, and did you do everything you could for them—forget those doubts. Put them behind you and keep celebrating your loved one's life. Remember the good times and let the bad ones drift away as subtly as a cool October wind.

You used to go to Mama when you had doubts and questions, even though you always acted like you didn't want or need her advice. It wasn't so much what she said, it was just that she was there, and now, you are no one's child.

You realize you are the oldest generation living and that is a little unnerving. You now face your own mortality and all that it represents. Even if your loved one was totally dependent on you, there was only the image in your mind that she was your parent. Every once in a while you could catch a glimpse of her smile, or disapproving eyebrows, that would send you back in your mind to when you were 12 years old. Your parent was the safety net you depended on and the only one in the world who loved you unconditionally. Now that is gone. At least in your mind it is.

When loved ones leave, we have a tendency to memorialize them. Somehow in our minds they become much bigger, smarter, and lovable than they really were. That's not a bad thing, unless you forget their humanity. They made mistakes, lost their tempers, and failed in some things in life, but that is what made them unique. If you look at your own attributes, you will find a lot of their traits in you.

You may no longer be anyone's child physically, but parents' spirits are alive forever, and they will never die. That is what the Bible promises us. Your Mama is still watching over you, and don't be surprised if she hasn't raised a few eyebrows about you moping around and mourning.

>>> **Your faith has been tested by fire and yet, here you are.** You are still reaching out to the Son of God, that fourth man in the fire who stood beside you when no one else was there. He promised you He would never leave you, and that was one promise Mama couldn't make.

What Mama could do was leave some of herself behind, and it is in those cardboard boxes. Now is the time to take what she has left behind and help those around you who are in need. And yes, other people are mourning the loss of her. Your children need you now. They have also lost someone who represented a strong foundation that now appears to be cracked. They are wondering who is going to help them catch ladybugs, bait their hooks, and make them their favorite macaroni and cheese. They wonder who will send them cards every year on their birthday, and they ache because Mama won't see them graduate.

>>> **They know what you've been going through and are concerned about you.** They feel helpless and want to help, but don't know how. You've distanced yourself from them through this ordeal, and you've been traveling a road without them. They're looking for you the way you used to be and afraid you might have changed. How can you alleviate some of the sorrow and loss they feel?

You can start by going through those boxes and picking out something special of Mama's they can have. Give them a piece of her life, so when they are missing her, they can pull out her old broach or necklace and touch it. Give them pictures of her they can bury in their drawers until they need to see her. Others are suffering also, and Mama is expecting you to be the strong one. After all, isn't that how she raised you?

So wipe those tears away, dust the soot off of your heart, and come forth into the newness of life that is waiting for you. You may have been in the fire for a while, but just like forest fires that burn away all of the undergrowth and fertilize the ground, their purpose is to make way for new life to sprout.

You may no longer be anyone's child, but you have progressed to the honored title of mother or father, matriarch or patriarch, of your family. Turn those tears into laughter and those mulligrubs into a celebration of Mama's life. As she stands in that great cloud of witnesses in heaven, let her be able to look down upon your life and be able to congratulate herself on a job well done. And you thought she was finished with you...not a chance...remember, she is alive forevermore!

<<< Crossroads >>>

What are your feelings about the outcome? Are you prepared, resigned, afraid?

Family Caregiver's Response
My mom is now 90 years old. In life we all face the same outcome—some sooner than others.

Was it worth the sacrifice and why?

Family Caregivers' Responses
Yes, because she is my mom. I know the time given can never be handed back to me, but I would not change anything. I could have done other things in life with that time, but I am glad I did not.

It is worth any sacrifice, my father was always was there for me, and I will not abandon him.

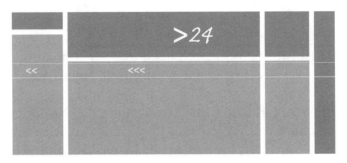

Two Dimensions, Two Journeys, One Destination

You Miss Their Essence

And I John saw the holy city, new Jerusalem, coming down from God out of heaven, prepared as a bride adorned for her husband. And I heard a great voice out of heaven saying, Behold, the tabernacle of God is with men, and he will dwell with them, and they shall be his people, and God himself shall be with them, and be their God. And God shall wipe away all tears from their eyes; and there shall be no more death, neither sorrow, nor crying, neither shall there be any more pain: for the former things are passed away. And he that sat upon the throne said, Behold, I make all things new. And he said unto me, Write: for these words are true and faithful.
—REVELATION 21:2–5

Mama is gone and each morning brings a new awareness of all you are going to miss. There will be no more phone calls, or hearing her special voice that could soothe your raging anger, chase away monsters hiding in the closet, and read the Scriptures as if they were spun gold. No more touching her fragile hands, the hands that felt your brow for fever, lovingly braided your hair, and tied your shoestrings. There will be no more sweet scent of lavender, yeast rising in the oven, or her clove-studded oranges at Christmastime. Your senses are starved for her presence and your heart is so heavy. What will tomorrow bring, and the day after that?

>>> **Isn't it awesome that you have so many precious memories of Mama to draw on?** You have been blessed, because many have never experienced a loving parent who showered them with kisses and encouraged them in all they did. Your Mama gave you the courage to go forth in life and be everything you could be, while at the same time she kept you close. Don't you wonder how she did it? How did she have the wisdom to get the formula just right? She may have been aggravating at times, but her love made up for it. How about all the unsolicited advice she gave you? Now you understand, it was just her concern for you. What you would give to have her aggravating you one more time. But that is not going to happen, and you know it. So what did Mama leave you that you have yet to discover?

If you look at your life, you can see the impact Mama made on it. See how you put the carrot in the spaghetti sauce to absorb the acid? That little trick came from Mama. How about your ability to throw a load of clothes in the washer, toss a chicken into the oven, all the while listening to your child's rendition of his or her day at school? Yes, that's what you observed...Mama multitasking.

Your journey in life began the day you were conceived. You have been able to reach heights you never thought you could because Mama was your support net. If you stumbled, messed up, or totally blew it, she was there to encourage you and point you in the right direction. You're no longer a child, and isn't it clever that no matter how old you got, Mama could set you straight with just a raised eyebrow or a whispered voice?

>>> **All her life she was preparing you for when she would no longer be here.** There was a reason she had you do a chore two or three times until it was done just right. She was challenging you to be the best she knew you could be. Mama was infusing you with the will to keep doing something until you got it right, and that's called stamina. How about when she made you fess up to a lie? She was building integrity and honor in you, a principled life, where you could always stand freely before the Lord.

Remember when Mama would make you take a gift to someone less fortunate at Christmas or put your precious penny into the offering plate? She was teaching you the gift of giving and receiving. And what about when she made you be extra nice to that child in school who was being ostracized? She was teaching you empathy.

>>> **Laugh a little now.** Think of how intricately Mama planned your life. And all along you thought you were so self-reliant. She was more than a mother, she

was a teacher, just as Christ. She used the moments she had with you to shape and mold you into the person you are today.

Even if you did not have a good relationship with your parents, you still have a multitude of blessings they have left you. If they weren't picture-perfect, then you can learn from their mistakes and thank them for saving you the heartache of making those same mistakes with your own children. Yes, there are blessings in everything, if you look for them.

We all have our own roads to travel, and some people are fortunate enough to have a loving parent to travel that road with them. Either way, we all live our lives with our spiritual eyes fixed on the same destination, heaven. This is the guarantee we have as Christians, that we will live forever with the ones we love. We may be separated from them for a while, but time is so short when compared to eternity.

Think on these things and you will understand that Mama has gone, but her presence has not. She is in everything you do. You may have her engaging smile, her loving eyes, or her warm heart. And let's get real here. You might have her temper, her great wit, or her phenomenal ability to mess up whatever you do, but that's all good. She is alive in you, just as your children carry the impression of you in everything they do.

For some people it may be remembering Mama's biscuits, others may daydream of fishing with Dad, and some may long to see Dad carve the turkey just one more time.

>>> **So how do you get over missing Mama?**

You don't. It's OK to miss her as long as you

recognize there is a time for mourning and a time for rejoicing. Mama is now spending her days with the King of kings, walking on streets of gold in her youthful beauty with no pain or tears. Could you think of a better place for her? If you had the chance, do you really think it would be fair to call her back? Has her diminished capacity and bedsore-ridden body already escaped your thoughts? No, Mama is basking in her final reward, and for that, you must rejoice. She is watching you and encouraging you to go on and live your life to the fullest you can.

She is going to be all right. How do I know that? Because the Word promises us that to be absent from the body is to be present with the Lord. Mama is walking and talking with Jesus. The One that gave her life now has her to Himself, and He's waited very patiently for her. She was yours for a while, but now she is back with her Maker.

Even through all this you still want Mama back, don't you? How can you do that? There is a way. Remember how you lovingly folded all her clothes as you packed them away? What about those boxes in the garage? Go back and look very closely, you might just find Mama's dog-eared recipe for her special biscuits.

Got it? Now get the mixing bowl, the flour, and the salt. See how she lives and breathes again through you? Mama's not baking biscuits anymore, but you are. I bet you can even hear her hushed voice, "Child...wash those hands before you touch my biscuits...you've got to stir it a little bit more...quit opening that oven door!"

<<< Crossroads >>>

What did you find is the most important thing in your relationship with your loved one, and what will you remember the most?

Family Caregiver's Response
All I know is that look on his face when he is lying in bed and looks up at me as I bend down to kiss his forehead and tell him good night. It is a look that is imprinted in my mind, and one I don't think I will ever lose, at least I hope I never do..

Contributors to

Finding Your Way: A Spiritual GPS for Caregivers

Joni Blake
Jackie Frugé
Greg Harford
Larry Harford
Vincent Hourigan
Mary Frances May
Edwin Pryor
Evelyn Rainey
Gus Reeves
Betty Jean Thornhill
Southland Suites

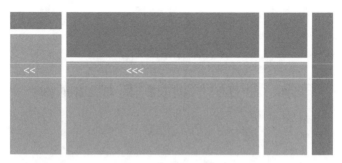

Additional Scriptures to Give You Direction and Clarity on Your Journey

I encourage you to read the whole chapter associated with each Scripture to not only understand God's acts . . . but also His ways.

Chapter 1 Anxiety

Be careful for nothing; but in every thing by prayer and supplication with thanksgiving let your requests be made known unto God. And the peace of God, which passeth all understanding, shall keep your hearts and minds through Christ Jesus.
—PHILIPPIANS 4:6–7

Take therefore no thought for the morrow: for the morrow shall take thought for the things of itself. Sufficient unto the day is the evil thereof.
—MATTHEW 6:34

Chapter 2 Responsibility

And went to him, and bound up his wounds, pouring in oil and wine, and set him on his own beast, and brought him to an inn, and took care of him.
—LUKE 10:34

Though I walk in the midst of trouble, thou wilt revive me: thou shalt stretch forth thine hand against the wrath of mine enemies, and thy right hand shall save me.
—PSALM 138:7

Chapter 3 Fear

For God is not unrighteous to forget your work and labour of love, which ye have shewed toward his name, in that ye have ministered to the saints, and do minister.
—HEBREWS 6:10

One thing have I desired of the LORD, that will I seek after; that I may dwell in the house of the LORD all the days of my life, to behold the beauty of the LORD, and to enquire in his temple.
—PSALM 27:4

Chapter 4 Discouragement

Behold, the LORD thy God hath set the land before thee: go up and possess it, as the LORD God of thy fathers hath said unto thee; fear not, neither be discouraged.
—DEUTERONOMY 1:21

But we have this treasure in earthen vessels, that the excellency of the power may be of God, and not of us. We are troubled on every side, yet not distressed; we are perplexed, but not in despair.
—2 Corinthians 4:7–8

Chapter 5 Loneliness

And I will come down and talk with thee there: and I will take of the spirit which is upon thee, and will put it upon them; and they shall bear the burden of the people with thee, that thou bear it not thyself alone.
—Numbers 11:17

And, behold, I am with thee, and will keep thee in all places whither thou goest, and will bring thee again into this land; for I will not leave thee, until I have done that which I have spoken to thee of.
—Genesis 28:15

Chapter 6 Patience

Then saith he to the disciple, Behold thy mother! And from that hour that disciple took her unto his own home.
—John 19:27

And Ruth said, Intreat me not to leave thee, or to return from following after thee: for whither thou goest, I will go; and where thou lodgest, I will lodge: thy people shall be my people, and thy God my God.
—Ruth 1:16

Chapter 7 Hope

Only take heed to thyself, and keep thy soul diligently, lest thou forget the things which thine eyes have seen, and lest they depart from thy heart all the days of thy life: but teach them thy sons, and thy sons' sons.
—Deuteronomy 4:9

Now we exhort you, brethren, warn them that are unruly, comfort the feebleminded, support the weak, be patient toward all men.
—1 Thessalonians 5:14

Chapter 8 Faith

But Nineveh is of old like a pool of water: yet they shall flee away. Stand, stand, shall they cry; but none shall look back.
—Nahum 2:8

And straightway the father of the child cried out, and said with tears, Lord, I believe; help thou mine unbelief.
—Mark 9:24

Chapter 9 Kindness

For his merciful kindness is great toward us: and the truth of the Lord endureth for ever. Praise ye the Lord.
—Psalm 117:2

Say to them that are of a fearful heart, Be strong, fear not: behold, your God will come with vengeance, even God with a recompence; he will come and save you.
—Isaiah 35:4

Chapter 10 Peace

Blessed are the peacemakers: for they shall be called the children of God.
—Matthew 5:9

Peace I leave with you, my peace I give unto you: not as the world giveth, give I unto you. Let not your heart be troubled, neither let it be afraid.
—John 14:27

Chapter 11 Guilt

For the flesh lusteth against the Spirit, and the Spirit against the flesh: and these are contrary the one to the other: so that ye cannot do the things that ye would.
—Galatians 5:17

Nevertheless there are good things found in thee, in that thou hast taken away the groves out of the land, and hast prepared thine heart to seek God.
—2 Chronicles 19:3

Chapter 12 Trust

Ye that fear the Lord, trust in the Lord: he is their help and their shield.
—Psalm 115:11

Then came she and worshipped him, saying, Lord, help me.
—MATTHEW 15:25

Chapter 13 Comfort

For the LORD shall comfort Zion: he will comfort all her waste places; and he will make her wilderness like Eden, and her desert like the garden of the LORD; joy and gladness shall be found therein, thanksgiving, and the voice of melody.
—ISAIAH 51:3

Blessed be God, even the Father of our Lord Jesus Christ, the Father of mercies, and the God of all comfort.
—2 CORINTHIANS 1:3

Chapter 14 Burdens

Thou wilt keep him in perfect peace, whose mind is stayed on thee: because he trusteth in thee.
—ISAIAH 26:3

Come unto me, all ye that labour and are heavy laden, and I will give you rest.
—MATTHEW 11:28

Chapter 15 Traditions

Therefore, brethren, stand fast, and hold the traditions which ye have been taught, whether by word, or our epistle.
—2 THESSALONIANS 2:15

And he took bread, and gave thanks, and brake it, and gave unto them, saying, This is my body which is given for you: this do in remembrance of me.
—Luke 22:19

Chapter 16 Financial Concerns

And I will give thee the treasures of darkness, and hidden riches of secret places, that thou mayest know that I, the Lord, which call thee by thy name, am the God of Israel.
—Isaiah 45:3

But thou shalt remember the Lord thy God: for it is he that giveth thee power to get wealth, that he may establish his covenant which he sware unto thy fathers, as it is this day.
—Deuteronomy 8:18

Chapter 17 Strength

Because thou shalt forget thy misery, and remember it as waters that pass away.
—Job 11:16

When his candle shined upon my head, and when by his light I walked through darkness;
As I was in the days of my youth, when the secret of God was upon my tabernacle;
When the Almighty was yet with me, when my children were about me.
—Job 29:3–5

Chapter 18 Instruction

Take fast hold of instruction; let her not go: keep her; for she is thy life.
—Proverbs 4:13

All scripture is given by inspiration of God, and is profitable for doctrine, for reproof, for correction, for instruction in righteousness.
—2 Timothy 3:16

Chapter 19 Praise

To appoint unto them that mourn in Zion, to give unto them beauty for ashes, the oil of joy for mourning, the garment of praise for the spirit of heaviness; that they might be called trees of righteousness, the planting of the Lord, that he might be glorified.
—Isaiah 61:3

The Lord is my strength and my shield; my heart trusted in him, and I am helped: therefore my heart greatly rejoiceth; and with my song will I praise him.
—Psalm 28:7

Chapter 20 Contentment

Who is as the wise man? and who knoweth the interpretation of a thing? a man's wisdom maketh his face to shine, and the boldness of his face shall be changed.
—Ecclesiastes 8:1

But we all, with open face beholding as in a glass the glory of the Lord, are changed into the same image from glory to glory, even as by the Spirit of the Lord.
—2 Corinthians 3:18

Chapter 21 Love

In a moment, in the twinkling of an eye, at the last trump: for the trumpet shall sound, and the dead shall be raised incorruptible, and we shall be changed.
1 Corinthians 15:52

Yea, though I walk through the valley of the shadow of death, I will fear no evil: for thou art with me; thy rod and thy staff they comfort me.
—Psalm 23:4

Chapter 22 Thankfulness

Thou hast granted me life and favour, and thy visitation hath preserved my spirit.
—Job 10:12

Thou wilt shew me the path of life: in thy presence is fullness of joy; at thy right hand there are pleasures for evermore.
—Psalm 16:11

Chapter 23 Joy

Therefore the redeemed of the Lord shall return, and come with singing unto Zion; and everlasting joy shall be upon their head: they shall obtain gladness and joy; and sorrow and mourning shall flee away.
—Isaiah 51:11

And ye now therefore have sorrow: but I will see you again, and your heart shall rejoice, and your joy no man taketh from you.
—John 16:22

Chapter 24 Heaven

And God shall wipe away all tears from their eyes; and there shall be no more death, neither sorrow, nor crying, neither shall there be any more pain: for the former things are passed away.
—Revelation 21:4

I will not leave you comfortless: I will come to you.
—John 14:18

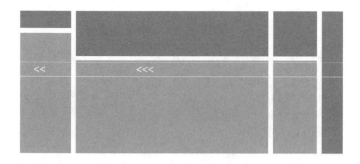

Resources for Caregivers

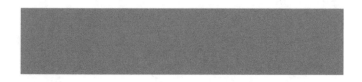

There are many resources out there for caregivers, so take advantage of them. I have listed a few below to get you started!

Administration on Aging—Offers a range of services to support family caregivers.
http://www.aoa.gov/AoARoot/AOA_Programs/HCLTC/Caregiver/index.aspx#purpose
Phone: (202) 619-0724

American Health Assistance Foundation—For help with Alzheimer's disease.
http://www.ahaf.org/
Phone: 1-800-437-2423

Caregivers4Seniors—Helps families find resources to care for their loved ones.
http://caregivers4seniors.com/
Phone: (808) 923-5918

Caring Connections—A program of the National Hospice and Palliative Care Organization, an initiative to improve care at the end of life.
http://www.caringinfo.org/
?gclid=CIOC49zU5KICFcpd2godkX6CIA
Phone: 1-800-658-8898

Eldercare Locator—To help you find local agencies to access home and community-based services like transportation, meals, home care and caregiver support services.
http://www.eldercare.gov/Eldercare.NET/Public/Home.aspx
Phone: 1-800-677-1116

Family Caregiver Alliance—A national caregiver's resource center.
http://www.caregiver.org/caregiver/jsp/home.jsp
Phone: 1-800-445-8106

Medicare.gov—Caregiver resource center.
http://www.medicare.gov/caregivers/
Phone: 1-800-Medicare

National Alliance for Caregiving—The alliance conducts research, does policy analysis, develops national programs, and increases public awareness of family caregiving issues.
http://www.caregiving.org/
Email: info@caregiving.org

National Family Caregivers Association—Educates, supports, and represents more than 65 million caregivers.
http://www.thefamilycaregiver.org/
Phone: 1-800-896-3650

Parkinson's Training for Caregivers—A free online course developed to train caregivers dealing with Parkinson's disease.
http://www.parkinsonseducator.org/

Senior.com—A Web site for baby boomer caregivers.
http://www.senior.com/caregivers/
Phone: (949) 713-1400

USA.gov—Find help for providing care, hospice locator, government benefits, legal matters, end-of-life issues, long-distance caregiving, support for caregivers.
http://www.usa.gov/Citizen/Topics/Health/caregivers.shtml
Phone: 1-800-333-4636

Online Caregivers' Forums

Alzheimer's Association Online Community—Talk with others dealing with caring for those with Alzheimer's patients.
http://alzheimers.infopop.cc/eve/forums/a/frm/f/214102241

CancerCompass—Empowering cancer patients to make informed decisions.
http://www.cancercompass.com/message-board/caregivers/1,0,122.htm

Caregiver.com—For Caregivers, About Caregivers, By Caregivers.
http://forum.caregiver.com/
Phone: 1-800-829-2734

Parkinson's Disease—Share your concerns with others.
http://www.myparkinsons.org/cgi-bin/forum/forum_show.pl/forum_show.pl

Journal Notes

Journal Notes

Journal Notes

Journal Notes

Journal Notes

New Hope® Publishers is a division of WMU®, an
international organization that challenges Christian
believers to understand and be radically involved in
God's mission. For more information about WMU,
go to www.wmu.com. More information about New Hope
books may be found at www.newhopepublishers.com.
New Hope books may be purchased
at your local bookstore.

If you've been blessed by this book, we would like to hear your story.
The publisher and author welcome your comments and suggestions at:
newhopereader@wmu.org.

Other resources for the "sandwich generation" by *New Hope Publishers*

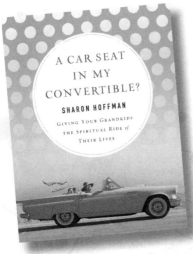

A Car Seat in My Convertible?
Giving Your Grandkids the Spiritual Ride of Their Lives
Sharon Hoffman
ISBN-10: 1-59669-208-1
ISBN-13: 978-1-59669-208-4

Coach Mom
7 Strategies for Organizing Your Family into an All-Star Team
Brenna Stull
ISBN-10: 1-59669-022-4
ISBN-13: 978-1-59669-022-6

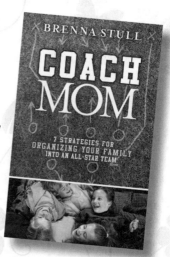

Available in bookstores everywhere.

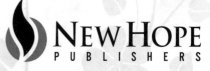

For information about these books or any New Hope product, visit www.newhopepublishers.com.